KU-654-234

NEURON

Smart Wellness Made Easy

Julia Jones, PhD
aka Dr Rock

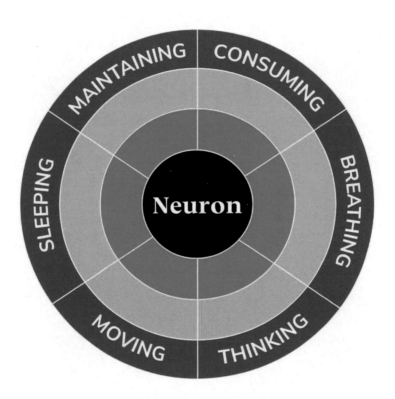

NEURON

CONTENTS

PART ONE
How & Why I Hacked My Health

PART TWO
My New Daily Habits

ACKNOWLEDGMENTS

My special thanks and gratitude to all the many family members, friends and colleagues along the way who helped make this book a reality. Extra special thanks to Rachel, mum, Sassy, Mark, Rufus, Charlie, Gia, the Devonshire Meirkats, Flossie and Mazza. In addition, there are many people in this field who have inspired me and continued to keep me motivated in this lifelong quest to discover the easiest route to a long, healthy life. Thanks also to James Drury for proof reading, Bob and Neil at This Day in Music Books for bringing this manuscript into their catalogue, Nigel and team at Biddles Books for printing, and Dominic Mohan for helping us reach audiences. I hope you enjoy the read and that some or all of the insights featured in this book help you transform your wellness in the way they've changed mine.

Disclaimer

The information in this book presents the science-based wellness techniques Julia embedded in her own life. They are not medical recommendations; they are educational content. As with any health-related activity, you should first consult with your doctor if you believe you may have any underlying health concerns that make some of these techniques inappropriate for you.

Definitions

Neuron
The amazing nerve cell that rules our existence

Biohacking
The purposeful use of specific techniques to optimise our natural biological functions, and consistently achieve wellness and high performance with ease

Music
One of the most versatile and effective biohacks at our disposal

Smart Wellness
(i) Learning about your evolutionary brain and body systems so you can look after yourself properly with informed choices and actions
(ii) The use of biohacks and technology to boost the above

Action Potential
(i) The electrical impulse that enables neurons to communicate chemically with each other
(ii) The mindset you'll hopefully unleash once you've read this book – recognising your potential to take action and enjoy a healthier, longer life

Preface

Ask yourself this question: why haven't decades of diet and fitness promotions and crazes produced a healthy population yet? They have entirely failed to achieve that goal despite billions of pounds/euros/dollars spent on persuading people to improve their nutrition and increase their exercise. In fact, over those decades, our health problems have skyrocketed so severely that they're deemed by many governments and the World Health Organisation to have reached crisis levels. Health and fitness revenues have steadily increased over the decades, but so has our average waistline size. Customers sign up for gym memberships, personal training courses, diet plans and buy home exercise equipment, but most struggle to sustain the effort. It's a great financial business model but not an effective long-term health solution. There are scientific reasons for this, and it involves our brain.

I don't believe that a continued focus on diet and fitness promotions will fix and futureproof the nation's health. This approach would have worked by now. This approach has failed because good health is determined by daily habits, decisions, choices and behaviours – the things powered by our brain and nervous system. Most diets and exercise regimes promoted to the general public do not align with our in-built and ancient brain and body biological circuits. So for most people, it takes a lot of mental effort to keep doing them. I believe we urgently need to start teaching everyone about their brain. That knowledge is more likely to lead to a lifetime of good health. I recently gave a short masterclass webinar for Wickes, a major UK retailer in the Do-It-Yourself home improvement sector. At the start of the session, I said: "*Good health is the ultimate DIY project.*" It's true. No-one can do it for you. It's something you have to take responsibility for yourself, and it's a project that lasts your entire lifetime.

To test my hypothesis, on 1 January 2020, I began a 12-month experiment on my brain. It was part of the research process for this book. I wanted to see what would happen if I took hold of my brain by embedding a range of biohacks into my daily routine.

Over 30 years, I've gathered a depth of knowledge and experience in neuroscience, psychology, and physiology as an academic and a practitioner. I've also been biohacking on and off since the 1990s. However, the results of this experiment still astounded me. My wellness scores have been supercharged. I've knocked several years off my biological age and extended my healthy life expectancy.

I've written this book to show you what I've learnt and how I did it.

Wellness is an art. In recent generations, we made many mistakes, yet those inaccuracies regarding health advice are still promoted today. We must disrupt our typical approach to health. It's out of date.

As well as the new things I learned, this experiment reminded me of the knowledge I'd amassed over the years but got out of the habit of embedding in my routines due to the chaotic nature of life. It's also reminded me of experiences that I'd forgotten, such as the afternoon I once spent with Richard Gere, the Dalai Lama and a room full of enthusiasts in New York in the 2000s, and the guidance I gave young Olympic hopefuls in the 1990s. All those sessions involved natural practices (now known as *biohacks*) such as breathing, music, gratitude and self-hypnosis. These are techniques that have long been taught as standard practice to elite athletes and monks to put them in control of specific brain circuits and nervous system responses, allowing them to enter and control different levels and states of consciousness. Things we previously could only measure with expensive equipment that I had access to in the lab are now accessible using affordable, readily available tech devices. These highly effective health practices are finally seeping into mainstream awareness and attracting increasing media attention, thanks in part to the rise of the new term *biohacking* in recent years, and the growing realisation that "we've got it wrong".

I first discovered these approaches in the early 1990s when, as a newly qualified tennis coach, I read the superb book *The Inner Game of Tennis* by Tim Gallwey. Shortly afterwards, I read my first music neuroscience research paper while studying psychology as an undergraduate. That was my eureka moment! I've been biohacking on and off ever since. Music has always been one of my 'go-to' brain- and body-hacks due to its versatility and fast-acting effectiveness.

Biohacks encompass many different interventions, but I only used natural ones for my experiment and this book. I didn't implant any cybernetic devices into my body or use supplements (apart from essential vitamins and minerals). I want this book to present straightforward, affordable techniques that everyone can adopt. I simply used natural interventions such as sound, vision, moving and breathing techniques that were likely to help my biological brain and body circuits function optimally. This means anyone can replicate them. You don't need expensive equipment or memberships.

Using simple biohacks embedded in my daily routines, my health scores went up, and my weight went down. I wasn't even trying to lose weight. It just happened as a natural side effect, driven by small changes in my daily behaviour. These hacks even managed to keep me on track when the Covid-19 pandemic hit, bringing business and family turmoil into my life with it.

I'll explain all the details throughout the book and share my journal notes, doodles and occasional setbacks. I'll also be exposing many of the health mistakes we now realise are glaringly apparent, yet still regularly appear in the news.

Good health is easier than we're led to believe (intentionally or unintentionally) by some business sectors, which still feed us misleading and outdated information. I hope the things you'll learn in this book will transform your approach to wellness forever. Read it, embed the habits into your own life, and pass the knowledge on to friends and family.

Chapter 1

Back to the Future

It's time to disrupt our typical approach to wellness because it clearly doesn't work

Firstly, let's set the scene and look at the status of the world right now. It's important to recognise the need to disrupt the current approaches to health and wellness because they haven't worked. The following pages outline some rather glum facts, but I promise you the rest of the book is full of good news. Excellent news, in fact.

It's become increasingly apparent that our very distant ancestors discovered many of "the answers" thousands of years ago. Then, in modern history, we buried all that wisdom under our attempts to "fix" human problems. The result? An unhealthy population, living in an increasingly polluted environment.

We thought we'd found the answers when we began inventing things like cars, light bulbs, and pharmaceutical medications, but it seems the real answers had already been discovered by our ancient relatives long ago. It turns out that we simply created more problems.

I've read close to 1,000 academic papers and books and devoured hundreds of hours of TED talks and lectures by the world's leading experts while researching this book. The scientific community has reached a consensus – we may live in a modern world, but we still have a very slow-to-evolve ancient and primitive brain that's wired for survival.

The answers were evident in the writings of our predecessors dating back thousands of years. If you want to master the art of good health, you have to master your brain. That's the route to lifelong wellness.

Your decisions, habits and behaviours dictate your health, and your brain flips those switches. This book pulls together the latest science and knowledge from across this broad field into one easy-to-follow guide. The good news is that lifelong wellness is a lot easier to achieve than you might think. We've been overcomplicating things. I started to present a lot of the science in my previous book, *The Music Diet*, because music is a highly effective biohack. It's been my tool of choice for boosting my performance and that of my clients for decades. This follow-up book takes an expanded view of health tools such as music and presents critical information about our brain, enabling you to broaden your approach to wellness, and giving you a programme of simple habits using proven tools, biohacks and shortcuts. I'll show you the fast-emerging field of smart wellness. We'll explore how technology and artificial intelligence are merging with brain science and biohacks to help us stay healthy - with a minimum of effort. Efficiency is the key. Unlike many of our previous inventions, these health tech innovations aren't trying to mess with, bypass, or outsmart our natural biological systems. They're designed to help us understand, monitor and activate them, allowing them to function naturally.

Get your hands on the steering wheel

The human brain is the most sophisticated structure in the known universe. It's still largely a mystery despite all we've learnt about it through decades of neuroscience research. Remarkably, we're each handed one of these powerful organs at birth. Yet most people aren't shown how it works, how to control it, and how to look after it, so it lasts a lifetime. I've always found this a little odd. It's like handing someone the key to a Formula 1 car without giving them any instruction. It's dangerous and likely to end in a crash. I've written this book to put you in the driving seat of your brain. Once your hands are firmly on the wheel, you'll more easily navigate your route to smart wellness.

Last year I randomly asked 100 people how much they knew about the brain. Over 90% of them responded with "very little" or "absolutely nothing". I've been asking this question since the 1990s, and the answers have typically been the same. We're not taught about our brains in school, so most adults never learn about it unless they actively seek that knowledge to boost their performance or health.

Thousands of years ago, the ancient Greeks made Apollo the god of music and medicine – things that we subsequently tried to prise apart, labelling them as distinctly different – i.e. *art* vs *science*. The opposite definitions can equally apply – music is a science, and good medicine is an art. The World Health Organisation now recognises the health value of music. Sound triggers myriad specific responses in the brain. Apollo was the god of sunlight, too, another natural wellness ingredient. The Greeks weren't the only people writing about these things back then. Early yogis also used chanting, sound, music, meditation, visualisation, natural light and breathing.

We seem to have lost our way a bit in recent generations. Our excitement about inventions got the better of us. However, I've noticed a distinct change in the past 18 months. The world is recognising and accepting that the so-called *solutions* we created caused unforeseen negative consequences that were often not evident until much later. The human race is now looking back into the past to find answers for our future health - answers that were there all along. Here's an example: why do you think music is present in every culture on the planet and is known to have been a part of human life for many tens of thousands of years? Why do you think babies and young children respond to music with singing, dancing and smiling? Why do you think we automatically make soft musical sounds with our voice when trying to soothe babies? These responses are witnessed globally across many different cultures. Is it a coincidence? Is it because it's entertainment? Is it because these responses are taught? No. Our human relationship to sound and music is unique and powerful. We'll explore this and many other things in later chapters.

The pandemic has amplified this growing shift in mindset regarding the search for the holy grail of wellness. In the last two years, the *New York Times* bestseller lists frequently feature books about aspects of the brain and nervous system, such as breathing, habit formation, and mindfulness. These topics also appear regularly in documentaries and print media.

Here's a simple fact: We need to stop what we're doing and go back to basics if we want to achieve lifelong wellness. We're living to 100 but in poor health. That's not the sort of future that I want to live through. I'm sure you don't either. There are many reasons why people are living longer, but in poor health. The more I researched, the more I realised I've also succumbed to many of these mistakes myself over the past decade. Life tends to become all-consuming, and good habits get easily side-lined if you're not paying attention. Now hurtling at lightning speed towards my 50th birthday this year, I'm keen to fix my habits and futureproof my wellness.

On the following pages, you'll find 20 recent realisations that became apparent to me during my research process. Some you might already be aware of, others you might not. We'll thoroughly explore and resolve all these and more together.

My Top 20 Realisations
(in no particular order)

Realisation 1

Our default approach of prescribing drugs to fix health problems produced other health consequences that needed additional medication. It's a negative spiral of chronic illness that many people get trapped in, leading to a lifetime of popping increasing numbers of pills to keep symptoms in check. This chronic poor health is also suffocating the medical system. The average age of a chronic health diagnosis is now the early 50s in the UK (even the late 40s in low-income groups), signalling the start of decades of declining health and increasing levels of prescription medications.

Realisation 2

Our labour-saving inventions and processed foods created invisible chronic inflammation in our bodies, food-related illnesses, impaired immune systems, and hastened muscle and brain tissue decline. These resulted in common ailments that we habitually cover up with prescribed medication. The overuse of antibiotics is also now recognised as a serious concern due to their impact on our gut microbiomes - key components in our immune system, and brain and body function.

Realisation 3

Our incorrect positioning of fat as the 'health villain' in previous decades drove the rise of sugar intake and the creation of its cheaper and deadly alternative – high fructose corn syrup. This is a sweetener, and it became used in almost all processed foods and drinks, even meat products. It's more potent than sugar and as addictive as illegal drugs (it triggers the same reward pathways in the brain). The low-fat, high carb (sugar) approach in recent decades fuelled the obesity, diabetes and heart disease epidemics. It screws up our finely-tuned insulin system, as we'll find out in later chapters. Our teeth didn't fare well with this diet either. It turns out that sugar is the villain, and fat is vital to our nutritional health. The UK Government introduced a successful Sugar Tax in 2018 to incentivise manufacturers to change their product recipes. But much more needs to be done to draw attention to the deadly effects of our sugar addiction. Recent science also shows that our brain shrinks as our waistlines grow, leading to further dangerous effects that progress invisibly for decades.

Realisation 4

Dieting and gyms haven't produced healthy nations because they're quite an unnatural thing for our brains to comprehend. So, most people have to force themselves into maintaining these inefficient, time-guzzling acts. These programmes and facilities can help achieve high fitness levels, ever-increasing personal best scores, and social contact, but they aren't necessary for simply maintaining basic wellness as you'll see in later chapters.

Realisation 5

Modern society confuses our ancient brain circuitry, which has evolved over millions of years to detect threats to our survival. As a result of this 'out-of-date operating system', the way we perceive stressful environments, such as a client deadline or work commute, can be misinterpreted by our brains as a predator or other threat to survival. This kicks off chemical chaos in our brains and bodies by triggering our 'fight or flight response'.

Realisation 6

Caesarean section births are now being linked to an increased prevalence of compromised gut microbiomes and immune systems in babies. They are also increasingly associated with an increased risk of other health problems, such as asthma and obesity. However, the findings are still somewhat contradictory at this stage until more long-term studies conclude.

Realisation 7

Bottle-feeding culture is now linked to the underdevelopment of babies' jaws. It increases the likelihood of crooked teeth and a lifetime of mouth-breathing and related health issues, such as asthma. Ancient skulls had straight teeth. It's believed the effort of drawing breast milk drove the full and broad development of the jaw. This was further enhanced by chewing actions before we started cooking and softening food. Our processed sugar habit wasn't a significant part of the human diet, so its damaging effects on teeth were not present.

Realisation 8

It appears that most people today do not breathe properly. Habitual mouth breathing is bad for your health. It exposes you to toxins and bacteria. These intruders are usually filtered before reaching the lungs if we bring air into our body through the route designed for breathing: the nose. The rise in gum disease and poor oral health (also driven by our addiction to sugar) is now linked to brain diseases, strokes and heart attacks due to bacteria in the mouth entering the bloodstream.

Realisation 9

Light bulbs and screens confuse our brain circuits, which assume it's sunlight. That screws up our sleep patterns and the quality of our sleep cycles. Sleep is an essential part of wellness. It's when our brain consolidates memories and cleans out toxins that have built up during the day. We don't get natural light in our eyes early enough in the morning, and we get artificial light in our eyes too late at night. This negative impact on our sleep quality each night accumulates into serious health impairment over time.

Realisation 10

Open plan office designs create environments that make it very difficult for our brain to focus. The resulting overwhelming struggle to stay on top of workload is now the leading cause of work-related stress and results in a multi-billion-dollar economic cost. Chronic stress also drives unhealthy eating habits, alcohol and drug consumption – and impaired sleep – in the working population. In-office restaurants have tried to boost employee wellness by offering healthy options. However, balanced meals placed alongside a wide range of unhealthy options still make it too hard for people to make the right food and drink choices. They end up overeating because food is free and readily available. The result is weight gain.

Realisation 11

Television viewing habits have increased and become highly engaged and intentional, driven by on-demand binge-watching of multi-episodes and seasons. This results in extended stints on the sofa, which is linked to an increased risk of cognitive decline. In contrast, our music habits have become less intentional and increasingly passive, driven by too much choice and availability and the rise of machine-generated playlists that we use as background audio wallpaper. Consequently, we're not drawing as much health value from music as we could be. It's an incredible wellness super-tool that our ancestors used extensively, but we're no longer fully benefiting from it.

Realisation 12

Longer working days (and commutes) result in early starts and late finishes, which have created daily eating habits that occur within a timeframe that begins too early and lasts too long. We break the 'fast' with our first meal of the day, but if our overnight non-eating window hasn't lasted long enough, our body hasn't had time to enter a fasted state. Our system is still using up the fuel we ate the night before. So, we're overconsuming and storing excess calories as fat. The breakfast cereal industry played a significant role in convincing us that we need to prioritise eating as soon as we wake up. The reality is that most of us don't need to do that. We should be delaying our first meal until later in the morning to give our system a long enough window to process the food from the day before and not store the excess as fat.

Realisation 13

Supermarkets conveniently put all our food in one place, but they're crammed full of mainly unnatural, processed products that we shouldn't be eating or drinking. This retail environment and its products purposefully exploit our ancient brain responses through marketing activities, packaging design and ingredients. They are designed to trigger our brain chemicals. Sending a human brain into a supermarket is like sending a drug addict into a crack den. Hardwired responses driven by automated chemical reactions in the brain make it very difficult to resist temptation. We've developed the habit of regularly popping into a supermarket for a small number of things on the way home from work, rather than less frequent weekly or fortnightly shops. Unsurprisingly, this routine results in us buying more items than we intended – and those extra items are usually unhealthy choices. The ease of access to and affordability of food has also made our portion sizes balloon. We're simply overconsuming. I'll show you how to break your dangerously addictive supermarket habit in later chapters.

Realisation 14

Checkout aisles in filling stations and supermarkets position incredibly unhealthy and highly addictive sugar-laden snacks all around us, which are specifically designed to trigger your brain's responses and make you reach out and take one while you're waiting. Yet, cigarettes are now placed behind a screen, so we can't see them and have to ask for them. This is irresponsible retailing. On 28 December 2020, during the final edit of this book, the UK Government announced it would put legislation in place to stop supermarkets promoting unhealthy goods in this way in their stores by 2022. This needs to be extended to include filling stations.

Realisation 15

High streets are now full of fast-food chains because these corporations are one of the few businesses that can afford the cost of being in a prime retail location these days. In addition, the recent rapid rise of delivery apps makes it easier and cheaper than ever to get unhealthy junk food delivered to your door at the mere press of a smartphone screen. The consequences of this new convenience food trend won't become visible for several years but will undoubtedly arise.

Realisation 16

Pesticides, created initially to help us boost crops, contaminate the plants and animals we consume and are now linked to various subsequent human health issues. Yet, in our hectic schedules, we often neglect to properly wash the things we consume before putting them in our bodies.

Realisation 17

Plastic inventions are ending up in the oceans, as microgranules in sea life. Therefore, they are in the fish we eat and also inside us. We are yet to see how this will damage us in the long term.

Realisation 18

The Royal Society of Public Health has now recognised social media habits as more addictive than smoking or alcohol. Like processed foods and drinks, these online social products use persuasion psychology, which is intended to trigger your evolutionary brain responses and make you want them. It seems like we're starting to replace our physical and social networks with digital ones. The World Health Organisation has warned that social isolation and loneliness are more damaging to health than smoking. As humans, we need to experience proper feelings of connection with other humans regularly. These in-person connections produce important chemical responses in our brain. Socialising is a vital part of human existence and a core part of wellness that is often overlooked. Video call platforms, such as Zoom, filled the gap during the pandemic lockdowns and social distancing rules, but they do not fully reproduce the equivalent biological effect of human social contact in physical environments.

Realisation 19

Our working life doesn't provide enough social connections any more. Many employees don't form a strong, close friendship with any work colleagues. The new shift to remote working will possibly exacerbate this erosion of workplace bonds unless employers work hard to build a strong company culture with regular and successful social programmes.

Realisation 20

Industrially polluted air and forest fires carry mercury that settles on our lakes, rivers and seas and is now in our fish in the toxic form of methylmercury. This has gained more media exposure in the last two years as several celebrities have been diagnosed with dangerously high levels of methylmercury in their blood due to a diet high in certain types of fish known to carry the poison. This issue is particularly dangerous for women who are pregnant.

The things we invent often seem to have a negative health consequence. It's not always immediate, but it appears to be somewhat inevitable.

The good news is that now we understand these hazards, we can start to protect ourselves from them and use our increased knowledge to sidestep them. I call it *smart wellness*. We're going to turn our attention back to our natural, ancient evolutionary processes. The human nervous system features incredible in-built maintenance systems, which are designed to keep all our organs functioning well. However, our inventions and resulting behaviours interfere with them and prevent them from doing their job. Being in control of your brain is vital in a world where you're consistently surrounded by things that have been designed to trigger your neural circuits and influence your decisions and behaviour. You need to keep your hands firmly on the wheel to combat them. If you don't know how your evolutionary brain circuits work, you're competing on an uneven playing field. Whereas, if you learn how your brain works, you're instantly at an advantage.

Back to Basics

It turns out that while we think we're modern and sophisticated, our brains are still the same as our ancient hunter-gatherer ancestors. So, a lot of research attention in recent years has focused on the remaining hunter-gatherer communities in remote parts of the world. It's become clear that common trends among such communities show they don't *exercise* as such, they're simply in motion more often than us throughout the day. They do sit down a lot, but in between those times, they are more physically active than us, moving around doing tasks and playing with children. These communities eat less than us (because we're overeating), but they eat well. They eat natural foods (including those containing sugar, such as honey) from the environment. This gives a daily intake of plant-based fruit and vegetable items with occasional meat and fish. Singing and dancing are commonplace. Not because they're taught to do so, but because it's a natural human act. However, if people from hunter-gatherer societies leave their natural habitat behind and relocate to urban areas, we frequently see the chronic illnesses driven by modern life and internal inflammation, just like the rest of the urban population.

Our brains constantly change throughout life. This malleability is called 'neuroplasticity', and it's what enables us to learn. It's what makes our brain so powerful. However, the underlying mechanisms do not change quickly. These circuits of neurons, and the chemicals that trigger them, evolved over many millions of years. So, it's unlikely they'll recognise and adapt to our modern inventions during our lifetime. That's why understanding how our brain works is key to achieving lifelong wellness. We have to work harder than ever to keep our brain on track when it misinterprets a piece of information from the external environment. The great news is that as humans, we have the incredible ability to take a step back, assess what's going on in our brain, and consciously do certain things to correct it when it flies off the road. The following chapters will show you how to use these biohacks to supercharge and futureproof your wellness.

My 12-month experiment changed my life (for the better), and I hope it'll prove useful to you too. I consider *smart wellness* to be a luscious combination of three things: knowledge, biohacks and technology. Our brains and bodies are like smartphones that still run a very old and outdated operating system. So it's necessary to produce upgrades and patches that fix or sidestep these bugs and errors, so we run smoothly.

Based on the general health of the population, it's likely that some, or all, of these facts apply to you right now. You're possibly eating too much of the wrong food at the wrong time every day; not drinking enough water; not breathing correctly; the receptors in your eye are probably not getting enough natural light at the right time; you're probably not getting the right type of sleep; not moving often enough; not spending enough time being 'present'; not fully enjoying your work; struggling to focus and learn and remember things quickly; maybe you're spending too much time digitally socialising and not enough time physically socialising, and you perhaps don't know much about your brain. This book will aim to help you fix all of these and more.

The field of neuroscience is one of the fastest advancing and exciting things happening on the planet right now, and it'll transform our future. The marriage of neuroscience and technology is already revolutionising healthcare by developing new techniques, interventions and treatments. As a lifelong neuroscience and psychology geek, I've been fascinated by the brain for decades, and it's fuelled my personal life as well as my professional career. There's no doubt that understanding how the brain works is key to better health and a better quality of life. Mental health has been wonderfully promoted over recent years, and that's great to see. Now I'd like to see brain health and brain control also enjoy similar attention. A greater understanding of the basic neural processes, and an insight into how to steer them, can bring more control over how we feel and the decisions we make. This is taught as standard practice in elite sport, but it should be for everyone. The following chapters will present insights and basic recommendations that can help transform your health forever.

I've arranged this book into two parts: Part One forms the main content. It focuses on the science and the wellness hacks that underpin the *Neuron*: Smart Wellness approach visualised in the model below.

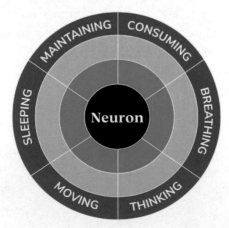

Part Two details the simple habits and hacks that I embedded into my daily routine as part of the experiment. These are the things that transformed my wellness over time with minimal effort.

By the end of the book, you'll have a good grasp of how the brain works and will understand that it's possible to have a lot more conscious control over it.

Chapter 2

A Quick Bit of Brain Science

Having a basic understanding of how your brain works instantly gives you an advantage when trying to achieve lifelong wellness

As mentioned in the introduction, the human brain is a phenomenal thing. The most sophisticated structure so far found in the known universe. We know a lot about it thanks to neuroscience advances, yet still know very little about it, due to its complexity. This chapter will give a simplified, yet comprehensive, overview of several important aspects of your brain.

We're all given one for free at birth, an amazing gift that we mostly take for granted unless it goes wrong. Think of what you could achieve in life if you actually knew how to operate this three-pound machine to its greater potential. There'll be a lot of information in the next few pages, but you're not going to be tested on it, so just try to absorb it and enjoy learning something new. The key thing you'll need to remember by the end of this chapter is:

There are certain evolutionary automated responses that get triggered in the brain, and YOU have the ability to exert control over them.

In terms of the history of our planet, we've been around a relatively short space of time. Homo sapiens have been on the earth for only about 200,000 to 300,000 years. And it's even more recently that we've been living with such high levels of interconnectivity and technology, meaning we're all still operating with a brain that was designed for a life of existence in a natural environment. Therein lies our problem. The brain is a highly sophisticated machine that operates in a dark, silent box (our skull). It assumes that the external information it receives through our senses is caused by natural stimuli, not the modern artificial inventions we've created in our modern society.

I know by now you may be chomping at the bit and wanting to get to the part where I show you the health hacks that I used. You'll get a lot more from the information presented in the rest of this book if you read this brain science bit, but if you really want to skip ahead, go for it. As a compromise, here's a quick summary of this chapter. Hopefully, you'll all read this bit.

- Your brain is made of 86-100 billion individual *neurons* (nerve cells).

- They communicate with each other using electrical impulses and chemicals. This happens day and night at super high speed for your entire life.

- Each neuron can have up to 30,000 connections with other neurons. This means our brain uses trillions of connections when it communicates.

- The electrical impulse travels from the main body of the neuron cell down a long projection to its end destination. This long arm is called the *axon*. The electrical impulse is called an *action potential*.

- When the electrical impulse reaches the end of the axon, a chemical is released. The chemical floats across a tiny gap before it connects with receptors on a nearby neuron. This area where neurons connect is called the *synapse*.

- Different chemicals do different things. For example, when dopamine is released and received by neurons in certain parts of the brain, it helps produce feelings of reward and motivation, encouraging us to keep doing an action (usually one our brain deems to be linked in some way to survival, such as eating). When glutamate is received, it excites and activates neurons, acting as an accelerator. When GABA is received, it acts as a brake, stopping neurons from activating. GABA is messed up a lot when we have a few alcoholic drinks. When cortisol is released, it helps move stored glucose into our bloodstream so it can be used as fuel, to provide a burst of energy. However, if too much cortisol is released for too long, it's damaging, and we associate it with chronic stress conditions.

- *Circuits* are collections of neurons that are highly connected and involved in certain tasks (e.g. memory). All our actions and experiences involve multiple circuits of neurons in lots of different regions around the brain.

- Some chemicals switch neurons on and off, to trigger activation. Other chemicals control whether the level of activation is high or low (they modulate the neurons).

- There are other cells that surround the neurons and are responsible for making sure the neurons are working well. These are known as *glial cells* and are highly important for keeping the environment around neurons clean and tidy.

- The outer part of our brain (the bit visible to you if you were looking at one) is known as the *cortex* and processes the masses of information that we're constantly receiving from the outside world via our senses. Thankfully, it decides which pieces of data we need to know about so we're not overwhelmed. It has four lobes. The front one (the frontal lobe) is what gives us an advantage over other species. The neurons there help us plan, make decisions, and communicate with other humans.

- Underneath that cortex layer, there are collections of neurons known as the *limbic system*. This is the emotional centre of our brain. It's highly connected with the information being processed by the cortex and our memories of past experiences. It also contains brain structures that play a crucial role in maintaining the wellness and operation of our brain and body systems.

- The lowest and evolutionarily 'oldest' part of our brain is the *brain stem* and an area called the *cerebellum*. These areas are involved in a huge array of subconscious processing of information important to our survival and emotional behaviour.

- Brains are constantly changing as connections between neurons are lost, and new ones are formed.

Brain tissue naturally declines throughout adulthood. Our muscle cells do too. However, just as we can stay strong by putting our muscles to work, we can also slow the decline of our brain tissue by putting those neurons to work and looking after them. We create new synapses throughout life when our brain does something new. It loves novelty. This constant rewiring of our brain, as some unused or damaged synapses are lost and new ones formed, is called *plasticity*.

• The brain and spinal cord are known as our *central nervous system*. Other branches of our nervous system exist and do other things. For example, the *peripheral nervous system* connects our central nervous system to our organs, limbs and skin so the brain can send instructions and receive feedback.

• Our *autonomic nervous system* is part of our peripheral nervous system and includes our flight or fight response. This system will come up a lot throughout this book because it plays a key role in how much we enjoy life or not.

• We have a vast team of internal systems that continually monitor and maintain our brain and body's wellness. The *hypothalamus* in the brain plays a key role in ensuring this ongoing *homeostasis* (a steady state of optimal functioning) by influencing our autonomic nervous system and directing hormone release throughout the body by triggering the *pituitary gland* that sits just outside of the brain. Modern society and the way we live today can get in the way of these systems and stop them from doing their job properly. Biohacking is highly focused on all these various natural systems, helping them to function optimally.

- Most importantly: unlike other creatures, we have the ability to think about, intervene, and adjust the signals that our brain is sending. Through training, we can also improve our ability to exert this level of control and train our brain to do what we want it to do. This is the key to lifelong wellness. We can use our knowledge and conscious control to stop habits that are damaging to our health and form new habits that enable our brain and body circuits to get on with the job of keeping us healthy.

If you'd like to explore further, here are 20 of my favourite brain structures and chemicals.

1. The (Amazing) Neuron and its Action Potential

The brain has 86-100 billion nerve cells, known as neurons. You can see a basic example of one I've doodled on the front cover of this book. Our neurons are responsible for making sense of our world and keeping us alive. They do this by passing chemicals to each other using electrically-charged signals (our brainwaves). Each neuron can be connected to other neurons by up to 30,000 receptors on their receiving protrusions (called dendrites), meaning the brain operates using hundreds of trillions of connections. Chemicals are received from other neurons via these receptors on the dendrites. If enough is received into the neuron's main cell body, an electrical signal, known as an action potential, is triggered along the long projection (the axon). When it reaches the end of the axon, chemicals are released across a gap called the synapse, or synaptic cleft. Those chemicals can then be received by dendrites of other nearby neurons and may also trigger a response in those nerve cells. This electrochemical chain of stimulation continues between neurons until the chemical response is no longer strong enough to activate the next neuron or the task has been completed (e.g. sending a signal to activate a specific muscle cell). Some chemicals are designed to activate the neuron, and some inhibit the effect and act as a brake. Our gut also houses a vast population of neurons and later chapters will discuss the increasing attention that nutrition is now being given in relation to mental health.

2. The Nervous System

Our nervous system comprises the central nervous system (CNS), which is the brain and spinal cord, and the peripheral nervous system (PNS) – a network of nerve fibres that branch out of the central nervous system, like a tree.

Our CNS features grey matter (the cell bodies and dendrites of the neurons) and white matter (the axons of the neurons look a different colour because they are coated in a fatty insulation that helps increase the speed of the electrical transmission).

There are also other cells around the neurons known as glial cells that play a supporting role in ensuring the neurons function properly. The brain consists of many regions, some of which we'll look at in the following pages. The spinal cord carries instructional messages from the brain to our muscles (known as motor signals) and receives information from our environment via our senses and relays it to the brain (sensory signals).

The PNS is divided into the somatic nervous system (handling voluntary movement and functions) and the autonomic nervous system (controlling involuntary functions).

We'll be discussing the ANS a lot throughout this book. It's responsible for our fight/flight/freeze response (the sympathetic branch of the ANS) and our rest/digest/repair response (the parasympathetic branch of the ANS). Maintaining control over your ANS so that your fight/flight mode doesn't dominate is a vital component of smart wellness.

3. The Autonomic Nervous System

This subdivision of the PNS plays a weighty role in how you experience life. It has enabled our species to survive and thrive. When it senses danger in your environment (or a general requirement for action), the sympathetic branch of the ANS triggers a fight/flight/freeze response – such as running away from an attacker. When this mode is not required, the other branch (the parasympathetic branch of our ANS) puts us back into rest/repair/digest mode so we can maintain our body and brain and be ready for the next survival emergency or action situation that requires rapid fuel. It's able to switch between these responses because it is connected via a network of nerve fibres to many of our internal organs, enabling it to dial up or down the activity of organs such as our heart, digestive tract, eyes. This brilliant system has kept us alive for millions of years. Unfortunately, it still thinks we're living in a natural environment and therefore sometimes gets thoroughly confused by modern inventions. A stressful day at work can trigger a fight/flight/freeze response, resulting in the release of stress chemicals. When this happens repeatedly, it can cause extensive damage to our body and brain cells. Many chronic illnesses are now linked to frequent and sustained activation of the sympathetic nervous system. The following chapters will show you how to ensure your parasympathetic nervous system acts as a brake, keeping your sympathetic nervous system in check except for when it's needed. The main nerve of the parasympathetic branch is called the *vagus nerve*. You'll see how to improve the tone of this nerve and the health of your autonomic nervous system using nutrition, breathing, visualisation and music in later chapters.

4. The Pre-Frontal Cortex

Human brains are divided into four lobes that play important roles in things such as vision, sensory processing and the motor activation of muscles. The frontal lobe sits at the front of the brain and, in evolutionary terms, is the most recent addition (although it is still millions of years old). It features an incredible region of neurons known as the pre-frontal cortex. This area's growth enabled us to develop highly sophisticated levels of planning, decision-making, social interaction, and thinking. It's connected to many other regions of the brain and can help us judge what's going on and make the best decisions based on the sensory information available to us and from memories of past experience.

It's also given us the ability to think about our thinking and exert will power (metacognition). This book will aim to give you the knowledge and understanding to really get a grip of your pre-frontal cortex and maximise its incredible power. You'll learn how to reduce distraction and increase focus to boost your achievements. You'll understand how the reward system in the brain can negatively impact the proper functioning of the pre-frontal cortex (such as being unable to resist choosing unhealthy foods even though you know they're harming you)

5. The Gut-Brain Axis

I cannot stress enough how important your eating and drinking habits are. Your brain and body simply cannot function properly if you're shoving crap food and drink items into your mouth every day. You're holding yourself back and causing immense damage to your internal organs that won't become visible until you're some way down the road of illness. Poor long-term eating habits are extremely dangerous and drive internal inflammation and they accelerate your ageing process.

In recent years, there's been a significant scientific focus on the now-recognised link between our gut and our brain. This two-way communication link (known as the gut-brain axis) means that the microbes in our gut can influence our brain health and function, and vice versa. Many mental health problems are now being linked to our nutritional habits. It used to be thought that mental issues resulted in gastrointestinal symptoms. Now we realise that often it's the other way around. The problem may actually originate in the gut due to poor diet. This means mental symptoms such as anxiety and depression could be triggered by compromised gut health. We'll explore this further later in the book.

What you eat influences your mood and your ability to think straight. So, aim to take action using the techniques in this book and fix your unhealthy nutritional habits out once and for all. They are holding you back from achieving your full potential and slowly killing you.

6. Our Salience Network

This large network of neurons plays a vital role in enabling regions such as the pre-frontal cortex to function optimally. The salience network acts as a switch, detecting and filtering information received from multiple sources and initiating responses by activating or deactivating relevant brain circuits. It toggles between switching to our daydreaming mode circuit (known as the default mode network) and task-focused mode circuit (known as the central executive network).

When our mind wanders, we know the neurons in our default mode network are active. Daydreaming is an essential brain activity. It enables us to internally process information, reflect on past events and think about future events. We're often in this mode when we're not required to focus hard on something. For example, you may have noticed while driving that you passed certain parts of the journey without conscious awareness of them. However, if something demanded your attention, your salience network would quickly pull you out of default mode network and activate your central executive network so you could focus on the immediate task (e.g. slowing down to avoid something on the road).

Learning how to exert more control over this salience network switch can help you maintain focus on something. It can also help boost your creativity by switching to the default mode network. We'll look at how to train and improve this system in later chapters.

7. *The Limbic System*

This collection of brain circuits (groups of connected neurons) buried in the centre of the brain plays a key role in our emotions. It consists of several brain regions, including the amygdala and hippocampus. Other areas include the thalamus (relaying sensory information to relevant brain areas), the hypothalamus (regulating thirst, hunger, temperature and hormones) and the basal ganglia (involved in movement, learning, habit formation and reward processing).

Throughout this book, we'll frequently refer to the amygdala and hippocampus. The amygdala drives emotional responses, especially fear, anxiety and anger. It also attaches emotional contexts to memories. It's particularly good at storing fearful memories, and this can lead to phobias and avoidance behaviour in later life. It's involved in the triggering of our fight/flight/freeze stress response. If sensory information received via the thalamus is perceived as a threat (based on previous knowledge and experience), a fear response will be activated. This is intended to keep us away from dangerous situations and keep us alive. However, in today's world, the amygdala can become hypersensitive, triggering anxiety responses for many life scenarios that we find stressful.

The hippocampus plays a central role in memory formation. It's possible to boost function in this region by regularly learning new tasks that make the brain build new connections between neurons. We'll explore how to master your limbic system in several chapters.

8. The Reticular Activating System

The reticular formation is a collection of ascending and descending nerve fibres in the brainstem. The descending projections mostly relay motor and sensory signals to the body. For instance, they give us the ability to suppress pain in a traumatic event or control movement or posture. The ascending fibres are also known as the reticular activating system and are responsible for distributing the brain chemicals that are essential for consciousness, wakefulness, alertness, vigilance and awareness.

The reticular activating system can determine what you notice in your environment, and this can produce powerful results. You may have heard of the Law of Attraction. When you set very clear and intense goals, you often find that 'coincidences' start to become noticeable and opportunities arise that you may find incredible to believe. It's likely that your brain is simply bringing them to your attention because they are linked with goals that you've consciously set. Suddenly you find things start to fall into place as more and more of these 'coincidences' start to appear. This is your reticular activating system filtering relevant information and bringing it to your attention via the various pathways where it delivers key neurochemicals to activate neurons. Later chapters will explore the power of goal-setting.

9. Mitochondria

I first learnt about mitochondria as a sports science undergraduate studying psychology and physiology. These amazing little organelles live in our cells, providing energy, so our cells continue to function and survive. Fuel is received by the mitochondria in the form of glucose from the food and drink we consume. It converts it into energy that the cell can use.

Mitochondria are the power plants inside our cells. We cannot survive without them. When we exercise, our muscles suddenly need a much higher amount of energy, and our mitochondria throw themselves at that task, rapidly converting fuels into energy for the muscle cells to use. We'll look at this in more detail in a later chapter. There are ways to boost and maintain your mitochondria throughout life.

These organelles don't just exist in muscle cells; they are also vital components of neurons. The brain uses a vast amount of energy, requiring a lot of oxygen and glucose (delivered via the blood) for the mitochondria to keep up with the demand for the fuel required by our neurons.

The efficiency and health of your mitochondria decline with age, and this can accelerate if you're not looking after yourself properly. It's vital to keep your inflammation low and your antioxidant intake up in order to keep neurons (and other cells in the body) clear of harmful toxins. We'll explore how to boost your mitochondria in more depth later.

10. The HPA Axis

The hypothalamus and pituitary gland (in the brain) and adrenal glands (on the kidneys) are connected. They work together to act as our stress response system. When we encounter a stressful situation, the sympathetic branch of our autonomic nervous system kicks into action. This triggers an increase in heart rate, and breathing and perspiration. These stress symptoms are initiated by the release of chemicals that we'll discuss later (epinephrine and norepinephrine). The hypothalamus detects these chemicals and activates the pituitary gland, which in turn activates the adrenal glands. This process is a chain of electrochemical messages. When the adrenal glands are notified of the situation, they release the chemical that we associate with stress – cortisol.

Cortisol enables the body to cope with a prolonged stressful situation. It delivers increased quantities of oxygen and glucose to cells that need it (such as muscles if you need to run for your life). But this system is intended to be activated infrequently and for relatively short periods of time. Today, the HPA axis is regularly and mistakenly activated by modern life situations that we perceive as stressful even though they're not life-threatening. This prolonged elevation of cortisol levels is now linked to many chronic illnesses such as type-2 diabetes, obesity and cardiovascular disease. We'll be exploring how to use hacks to regulate your HPA axis and keep your cortisol levels under control.

11. Glutamate & GABA

These two chemicals are widespread in the brain. They are known as neurotransmitters and act as either an accelerator or a brake when received by neurons.

Glutamate is the accelerator. When it's received by receptors on the dendrites of neurons, it excites the cell. In sufficient quantities, it can trigger an action potential. This sends the electrical signal along the axon so it releases chemicals that can be received by the next nearby neuron.

GABA is the brake. When it is received by receptors on the dendrites of neurons, the cell is inhibited, making it less likely that an action potential will be triggered along the axon. This effectively stops the activity in that neuron (and the nearby neurons).

These two neurotransmitters work together in a fine balance to control our actions, thoughts and behaviour. Disruption in these chemicals can lead to overstimulation or under-stimulation of neurons in several brain regions. Our lifestyle can impact the normal operation of this pair. For example, alcohol significantly disturbs the status quo.

12. Dopamine & Serotonin

These neurochemicals modulate neuron activity in several brain regions and are known to play a key role in our mood, behaviour and attention.

Dopamine is designed to help us continue the effort to achieve things that are vital for survival, such as eating, drinking water and sex. This chemical isn't just released when we succeed and receive our reward; it's also released during the effort journey in order to encourage us to continue until we succeed. Dopamine is delivered via pathways from the midbrain to several brain regions known as our reward circuits. These circuits can be dramatically altered by drugs that mimic the effects of dopamine or by increasing the amount of dopamine that's available to receptors on neurons in reward centre regions of the brain. Either way, the result is that we feel good. This can lead to addictive behaviours whereby we want more and more of this substance (e.g. food, alcohol, prescription and non-prescription drugs). Eventually, they no longer have the effect we seek because the reward circuit is disrupted, and some receptors are damaged or lost. We then need more and more of the substance to feel an effect.

Serotonin is also associated with our mood and emotion and is commonly linked with depression. Prescription drugs purposefully aim to block certain channels to maintain higher levels of serotonin available to neurons.

We'll look at how to naturally maintain healthy levels of these neurochemicals later.

13. BDNF

Brain-Derived Neurotrophic Factor (BDNF) is related to the growth, maintenance and survival of neurons. It also plays a key role in learning and memory and is found in high levels in neurons in the brain's hippocampus region. Ageing and ongoing exposure to chronic stress can reduce levels of BDNF. As neurons die, this loss of grey matter can be seen on brain scans. Even before the neuron dies, it will gradually lose its ability to communicate with other cells. This is often noticeable and known as cognitive decline, whereby we may struggle with certain tasks and recalling or forming memories.

Your brain is constantly changing, enabling you to learn and remember things. This malleability is known as brain plasticity. However, these changes can be negative (when neuron function declines) or positive (when neurons thrive). To attain and maintain wellness through life, it's important to ensure we take steps to boost positive plasticity. We can do this by ensuring BDNF levels are healthy and by engaging in activities that tax our brain and require it to form new complex connections through novel tasks.

In later chapters, we'll explore how to maintain healthy levels of BDNF by improving your nutritional habits, increasing your physical activity and keeping stress at bay.

14. Acetylcholine

Another chemical involved in learning and memory formation is acetylcholine.

It's a key neurotransmitter of the parasympathetic branch of our autonomic nervous system, released and received in multiple areas of the body, activating smooth muscle tissue of internal organs to slow heart rate, dilate blood vessels and boost digestion. It activates the rest/digest/repair activity regulated by the parasympathetic nervous system.

Acetylcholine also stimulates our skeletal muscles to generate movement. When an electrical impulse reaches the end of nerve fibres and reaches a muscle fibre, acetylcholine is released and passed across to activate the muscle. It binds to the receptor on the outside of the muscle fibre.

Acetylcholine also plays a leading role in attention. Its activity on neurons in our pre-frontal cortex helps us to detect relevant cues in our environment and block out other distractions. This ability to keep informational "noise" at bay enables us to maintain focus on things we want to keep our attention on. Needless to say, this ability boosts learning and memory.

15. Oxytocin

Oxytocin is produced by the hypothalamus and released by the pituitary gland in the brain. It's known as the 'love chemical' and is boosted during reproductive behaviour. It is important for the stimulation of emotional responses and our positive social behaviour towards others. It helps us form bonds with family and friends and has been essential in community-building throughout human evolution. It enables us to trust others and create positive memories, and promotes bonding between mother and child. As well as enhancing empathy, it can also reduce the activation of the amygdala. This reduces our feelings of fear or anxiety.

Oxytocin is released when you are bonding socially with someone or in physical contact with a person. Therefore, being around others maintains a regular dose of this chemical. Our relationship with pets also gives us an oxytocin boost. Low oxytocin can increase our stress and make us feel less connected to others. This deficiency has also been linked to anxiety and symptoms of depression.

The World Health Organisation has officially marked loneliness as one of the most serious epidemics of our time, more damaging to health than smoking. Staying socially active throughout life is vitally important, especially as we age. Many older adults now live alone, with family members living long distances away. Staying social is even more difficult if the person is no longer physically mobile. Very strong emotional connections and attention is known to be associated with oxytocin release. Just being in a room with someone while fiddling with your phone won't work.

16. Cortisol, Adrenaline & Noradrenaline

Cortisol is well-known for being our stress chemical. Having this chemical constantly flowing at high levels is not good for us. It can cause a lot of damage and lead to many chronic illnesses. When we are chronically stressed, the sympathetic branch of our autonomic nervous system triggers the release of cortisol. So, keeping this under control is vital for wellness. Cortisol is not all bad, though. We need it to maintain our daily rhythm and sleep patterns. Levels of it rise in the morning to give us the boost we need to get our day going, and they should naturally be lower at night to enable us to go to sleep and rest.

Adrenaline is also known as epinephrine, and noradrenaline is also known as norepinephrine. They are both released by our adrenal glands when the sympathetic branch of our autonomic nervous system (fight/flight/freeze) is activated. This enables us to respond to the stressful stimuli we've encountered (or something we have perceived as stressful). We get a surge of adrenaline, and all the symptoms of our fight or flight response kick in, such as increased heart rate.

Aside from its role in our stress response, norepinephrine also plays other important roles, such as in our ability to maintain attention. Its presence in several brain regions and its interaction with other chemicals such as dopamine and serotonin help us to maintain effort and focus. So, it's important for us to have a certain level of arousal in order to function properly. However, when that arousal is too high for too long, it's detrimental.

17. Glucose, Insulin & Cholesterol

Glucose is the vital energy source used by the cells in our brain and body. It's delivered in our blood, and if levels become too high or too low, it can be fatal. Cells receive glucose from the food and drink we consume, and when that runs out, the body releases more of it from places it's been previously stored. Insulin plays an essential role in this because it's required to transport glucose from the blood into the cell for use as energy. If insulin isn't present, glucose builds up in the bloodstream and the cell is unable to access its fuel supply. Cells can become resistant to insulin if it's released too frequently due to your diet being overloaded with sugar and carbohydrates. This leads to type-2 diabetes. It's important not to overconsume sugars and carbohydrates. If not burned by our cells, excess glucose gets converted and stored as fat. It only gets converted back into glucose and into the bloodstream if the available glucose (from recent meals) and the first choice stores (glucose previously stored as glycogen in our liver and muscles) have been used up. So, if you're trying to reduce your excess fat stores, it's essential to minimise your intake of sugar and carbs to keep your blood glucose levels low enough to trigger the fat cells. We'll look at this in detail in later chapters.

Cholesterol also circulates in our blood and plays a role in cell health. However, it can build up as a dangerous waxy substance and cause cardiovascular problems.

18. Leptin and Ghrelin

Earlier, we looked at the neurotransmitters, GABA and glutamate, the 'stop' and 'go' chemicals that activate or deactivate neurons. Well, leptin and ghrelin are the 'stop' and 'go' chemicals that control our appetite and our eating and drinking activity. The recent obesity epidemic has sparked heightened scientific interest in this duo. When the healthy operation of ghrelin and leptin are disrupted, overeating and excess fat storage can arise. This increases the risk of weight-related diseases such as type-2 diabetes, cardiovascular disease, brain shrinkage and some cancers.

Ghrelin stimulates our appetite. It's produced in our gut when our receptors sense a lack of food there. It travels in the blood to our hypothalamus. Once the neurons in the hypothalamus receive this signal, we experience an urge to seek and consume food. Leptin signals to us that we have sufficient supplies and no longer need to seek and consume food. It's released from fat cells and, like ghrelin, it also signals to the hypothalamus to modulate our eating behaviour. If fat stores increase due to overconsumption, leptin also increases. However, this does not necessarily increase the effect of leptin and decrease hunger because leptin resistance can occur. In this instance, similarly to insulin resistance, the presence of leptin becomes ineffective, and overconsumption may continue. The precise mechanics of this process are still being understood.

19. Melatonin

Melatonin is produced in the pineal gland and is central to the maintenance of our sleep cycle. It's influenced by information from our external environment received via our eyes. When those visual receptors sense reducing light, they signal the release of melatonin. Therefore, levels are highest at night. This daily cycle is our Circadian Rhythm, a natural clock involving a region of the brain called the suprachiasmatic nuclei (a great name for a band, I think). Based on the light signals received during the day, this region inhibits the pineal gland to reduce the release of melatonin. As the light dims, this inhibition reduces, allowing the pineal gland to release more melatonin and putting us into sleep mode.

Many of us regularly disrupt this natural rhythm by exposing our eyes to bright lights at night and by not getting enough natural light when we wake up in the morning. Remember, our brain is still running a very old operating system. It doesn't know the difference between light from bright overhead lamps or a mobile phone, and that of natural light from outdoors. Melatonin production tends to decline in later life. This makes it harder for older adults to get sufficient good quality sleep. So, it's important to ensure that you're embedding good habits that maximise the sleep process. We'll look at this in more detail later.

20. O2, CO2 & Nitric Oxide

You already know about oxygen and carbon dioxide in relation to breathing. These gases are key players when it comes to keeping our cells supplied and healthy.

Oxygen enters our blood via the lungs and is pumped by the heart to all the cells in the brain and body. On its journey from the nose to the lungs, it is filtered, warmed and moistened in order to help it pass through into the blood. Earlier, we talked about mitochondria's role in converting glucose into fuel energy that our cells can use. Mitochondria also need fuel to complete that task, and that arrives in the form of oxygen. Carbon dioxide is a toxic waste gas produced by mitochondria in this process. It is transported back out of the cell into the bloodstream and carried back to the lungs, where it is expelled when we exhale.

Nitric oxide hasn't received as much attention as oxygen and carbon dioxide but is also a vital gas in the respiration process. The sinuses in our nasal cavities are one site of significant nitric oxide production. This means that the air we breathe in through our nose picks up this gas and transports it into the blood together with oxygen. It's a vasodilator, meaning that it acts on blood vessels of the cardiovascular system, relaxing and widening them to increase blood flow and lower blood pressure. If you're a habitual mouth-breather, you're missing out on this process.

PART ONE

How & Why I Hacked My Health

Using the
Neuron
Smart Wellness
Approach

Chapter 3

Consuming

Weight gain and obesity are now a global health crisis. They are also driving other related illnesses – but they're preventable

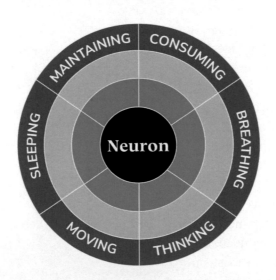

If you've ever tried counting calories to lose weight, you'll be aware that it can be a pain in the ass. As well as being annoying and tedious, it can accidentally lead to an avoidance of healthy foods because they're incorrectly considered 'calorific'. It can also sometimes push people towards processed foods because the packaging displays the calorie content for you, making it easier to log. Attempting to understand nutrition can be a confusing and miserable experience for most people, but here's the bottom line: you are what you eat. The molecules of food that enter your mouth instantly trigger myriad chemical reactions. Some of the food molecules eventually become new tissue within your body; some are converted into other chemicals that your body and brain use as energy or as messengers to trigger moods and behaviours; some create inflammation and destruction in your body. So, think very carefully about what you consume.

Eating has become a leisure pursuit in recent years — an entertaining, pleasurable hobby rather than a vital function for human existence. Television schedules are full of cooking shows and celebrity chefs tempting us with mostly unhealthy recipes. Eating and drinking can become an extreme sport if you abuse it and frequently engage in high-risk consumption habits. This chapter will examine our relationship with food and drink and review some tips on identifying and avoiding the hazards that surround us every day.

It's not just what we eat that impacts us. The timing and quantity of food also matter. Our systems are designed to exist on a relatively low amount of food. I remember when collecting my chocolate Labrador puppy from the breeder, a vet. He asked me how much food I thought a chocolate Labrador would need each day. I measured out what I thought was an appropriate amount, but he reduced it by half to just one measly looking orange beaker of dog food. This seemed like a tiny amount, but sure enough, it's been sufficient to maintain Rufus' healthy weight for the past nine years. Rufus still bounces around like a puppy even though he's now approaching 10 years old. That food contains all the nutrients he needs.

Food is our energy intake, and physical movement (plus our core internal processes) is our energy expenditure. Just like Rufus, our human bodies also do not need as much food as we think they do. When the energy from the most recent meal we consumed is used up, our biological systems simply source more energy from our internal storage units (food molecules we held onto from previous meals, kept as fat). This only happens when we're in a fasted state, when our stomach and digestive pipes have no usable food molecules left in them, and therefore, the fuel in our bloodstream runs out. In today's society, many of us never really enter that fasted state because we're eating too close to bedtime and then eating again as soon as we wake up. Plus, our portion sizes are far too large. Rather than our body using up excess energy reserves, we're constantly storing daily surplus energy reserves as fat. Let's look at how we got here.

In previous chapters, we saw that human brains still use the same circuits and responses that are wired for survival. They don't realise we now have easy access to large amounts of food. Sometimes our ancestors ate well, and sometimes they would have long periods where they could not find sufficient food.

Let's look again at the two hormones specifically related to our eating habits – ghrelin and leptin (the 'dining duo'). These ancient chemical systems work together to instruct brain circuits and body organs to regulate our appetite. The current obesity crisis led to a lot of research on these hormones over the past decade. These studies continue to see how humans might artificially manipulate these hormones to achieve weight loss. However, we're simply going to look at the fundamental way they operate in a natural state. This will help you understand how your appetite works and how to get in control of it.

Ghrelin is our hunger hormone. It's secreted by our digestive system when it is approaching empty. It tells the brain that we soon need to find and eat some food. After we've put food into our stomach, it decreases until the food runs out again and more ghrelin is secreted. It's thought that eating fewer, but larger meals is advisable because it means ghrelin is secreted less frequently (as it takes longer to digest a larger meal). In contrast, regular snacking throughout the day means the stomach is secreting ghrelin more often whenever the small snack is digested, and the stomach becomes empty.

Leptin has the opposite effect to ghrelin – it suppresses hunger. It's secreted by fat cells and tells the hypothalamus in the brain that energy is available to burn. This gives permission to fire up our metabolism and activate processes that require energy. By contrast, when energy is not available (and the hypothalamus is not receiving the leptin signal), our metabolism is dialled down to conserve energy.

Both these chemical signals talk to areas in the brain linked to metabolism and maintaining our healthy functioning (hypothalamus), reward behaviours (limbic system), our memories (hippocampus) and decision-making regions (pre-frontal cortex). Keeping your hormones balanced and in check is essential. You can see from the involvement of our reward pathways in the brain that we can quickly get into a situation where we're eating food items simply because they trigger the release of dopamine and strengthen that habit, and not because our body needs more food for survival. If you're gaining weight, the system is not working correctly, and you need to hack it and bring it back in line.

The Mighty Microbiome

Scientific research advances relating to our microbiome have leapt forward in recent years thanks to technology. The ability to conduct detailed genetic analyses has delivered a deeper understanding of the importance of this vast colony of approximately 100 trillion microbes inside our body and on our skin that call us' host'. The majority of them live in our gut, and we now know they are linked to a substantial range of health factors. Our microbiome make-up is unique to us and now considered an organ in its own right, due to the important role it plays in vital mechanisms within our body. We also know there's a critical connection between our gut and our brain. Our microbiome is involved in the synthesis of vitamins, the production of short-chain fatty acids for energy metabolism, immune system functioning, and it influences our behaviour by modulating various brain circuits. We cannot function optimally if our microbiome is compromised. So the food and drink we consume are even more vital than we once thought.

It all seems like a great system, so what the heck went wrong?

Our brain and body have many incredible in-built systems to ensure we remain healthy. However, when it comes to nutrition, humans made a mistake a few decades ago. Fat was described as a villain and the culprit of weight gain. Everyone jumped on this bandwagon, even national health organisations. The result was dramatic and rolled on for generations before we realised the mistake.

Now we know that fat is not the culprit; it's sugar. But by the time we figured this out, the food industry had showered us with 'low-fat' products and invented an endless alternative range of new carbohydrate- and sugar-laden or sweetener-fuelled products with which to fill our shopping trolleys. They pushed out our desire for fruit and vegetables, and the contents of our plates became increasingly beige. It turns out that not only is sugar linked with several adverse health effects, it's also highly addictive because it triggers the dopamine powered reward pathways in our brain. Food and drink manufacturers use sugar (both processed and natural versions) to activate your evolutionary circuits, making you want (and then need) their products.

Why is sugar so bad?

It's actually processed sugar that impacts us in particularly harmful ways. Our ancestors enjoyed – and today's hunter-gatherer tribes enjoy – sugar in their diet but from natural sources like fruits and honey, not the synthesised cheaper versions that we invented.

Our brain and body respond in a variety of ways when we consume too much sugar. Insulin, a hormone made in our pancreas, is a key player. It has many roles. When all is well, and our systems are working optimally, insulin is released by the pancreas when sugar levels are detected in the blood. This hormone is vital to help transport the glucose (sugar) from your blood into your cells so they can use it as energy. If there is more glucose present in the bloodstream than required for energy, insulin also helps take it to our muscles and liver, where it is stored as glycogen and kept in reserve until we need extra energy later. However, we now live in a world where our sugar intake (including carbohydrates that our body converts to sugar) has become immense. We consume far more sugar than we need for energy. This means that our glycogen stores become full and the remaining glucose circulating in the bloodstream is converted and stored in fat cells.

Frequent sugar intake and the resulting high levels of sugar circulating in our blood mean that the pancreas regularly secrets insulin to deal with it. It tells fat cells to hold onto their stores because they are not required to be released for energy due to the system's continuous availability of glucose. It inhibits fat breakdown. Overconsumption of sugar eventually leads to cells becoming resistant to it. This leaves sugar floating around in our bloodstream because insulin can no longer unlock cells to take it in for energy. Sensing the rising levels of sugar in the blood, the pancreas keeps releasing insulin, but the cells are no longer responding. This leads to damaging inflammation and dangerous consequences for brain and body tissue.

You could be insulin resistant for years before the symptoms become noticeable as the onset of type-2 diabetes. It's silent and deadly, but if your weight is going up, you could be on this course. Weight gain is a sign that your fat cells are not required to empty their energy stores into the bloodstream, or that too much sugar is already circulating and being stored as fat because it can't be used as energy. Either way, it's bad news and utterly messes up the balanced operation of your metabolism. To make matters worse, sugar can also mess up your cholesterol levels. This increases the risk of damage to the cardiovascular system and the lining of blood vessels even further.

How can you fix and future-proof your health?

Now you know that processed sugar is a serious issue in our society, and you know its biological reasons. It's time to reduce your intake and rebalance your daily nutritional habits. Remember: sugar exists not only in its natural form and fake processed alternative but also in the form of carbohydrates (because those are also converted to sugar by our body). This knowledge will help you avoid sugary foods. However, the additional problem is that sugar is highly addictive, especially the more potent, fake versions of sugar that were invented. It's possible that, at some level, you are already addicted to sugar. Your reward circuits in your brain have been enjoying the dopamine hit for years, and they have formed strong associations. Annoying, right? So, to reduce your sugar and carb intake, and replace it with natural plant-based fruit and veg items and proteins, you have to recognise your likely addiction to sugar and break the habit. We'll look at this in more detail later.

However, please don't think that a reduced sugar and carbohydrate intake is the answer. The answer lies in balance. We need some healthy fats, and we need some healthy sugars every day. The problem is that we are overconsuming unhealthy fats and sugars. Eat less, and eat well.

Animal fats are now linked with serious diseases. Red meat is classified as group 2, which means it 'probably causes cancer'. Processed meat is officially listed as a group 1 carcinogen known to cause cancer. Other group 1 carcinogens include mustard gas, tobacco and asbestos! There are even questions about the health values of fish and white meat due to toxins related to their production. So, ensure your daily intake is primarily dominated by plant-based foods (preferably organic to avoid pesticide intake) and large quantities of vegetables. Pile your vegetables onto your plate, and then add some more.

The Science of Alcohol

Alcohol intake has been a cause of concern in recent years. It's listed as a group 1 carcinogen. However, the evidence published in the media often presents a confusing and contradicting range of opinions regarding whether or not it's good for us. I doubt in the near future we're all going to give up alcohol. I don't intend to. However, it's helpful to know what happens when you consume alcohol. First, let's look at the effects on the brain. In the previous chapter, we looked at some brain science and examined how neurons communicate with each other using electrical impulses (the action potential) and then pass chemicals to each other via receptors located on the membrane of other nearby neurons. Two of the chemicals we looked at were glutamate (the brain's 'go' chemical) and GABA (the brain's 'stop' chemical). These work together to maintain a balanced system. Alcohol affects many types of receptors on neurons in several brain regions. This means it produces a wide range of noticeable changes in thinking and behaviour. Alcohol boosts GABA levels and activity, and this is one of the first changes we will start to notice. It starts to make us relaxed, then sleepy, as our excited neurons are gradually halted by increasing GABA. Alcohol also blocks the receptors that accept glutamate, reducing the activity of neurons. When this happens in the decision-making and judgement brain regions in the frontal cortex, we make bad choices and struggle to exert self-control. One drink after work turns into several, and then often ends up in a search for junk food on the way home. When our memory circuits shut down, we have no future recollection of the alcohol-fuelled experience. If GABA levels rise further due to a more alcohol intake, we eventually lose consciousness as more neurons across the brain become switched off.

It's not just GABA and glutamate that are affected by rising levels of alcohol circulating inside us. Serotonin, dopamine and endorphin effects in the brain are also enhanced. This results in behaviour we don't typically display. It can result in drawling out "I love youuuuuu" to strangers and dancing energetically on top of table-tops. Alcohol also triggers the dopamine reward system. This can lead to addiction.

Of course, it's not just the brain that suffers; alcohol impacts our entire body. It's effectively a toxic intruder, so our inflammatory response is activated once it's detected in our system. This is designed to protect our internal tissues and organs from damage. However, it's meant to be a temporary immune response. Frequent and ongoing inflammation is harmful and now linked with several chronic diseases such as cancer and diabetes. Alcohol destabilises your finely balanced brain chemicals and systems. It should be enjoyed in moderation. The new rise in low alcohol and no alcohol drinks will hopefully help us transition out of the extraordinarily boozy habit we've begun to consider as normal in society.

Food and Mood

In the previous chapter, I mentioned the gut-brain axis. The food and drink you consume can affect your finely balanced brain and body circuits as much as the pharmaceutical drugs you are prescribed. Health issues that used to be considered a cause of gut problems are now considered a symptom of gut problems. Many of these mental health issues actually originate in the gut and can be significantly influenced by a change of diet. The gut bacteria that make up our microbiome play a vital role in producing key brain chemicals such as serotonin, dopamine, glutamate and GABA.

Depression is now linked with overconsumption of sugar. Sufferers can find themselves trapped in a complex spiral as their cravings for sweet rewards intensify and high sugar foods become used as a comfort. Many carbohydrates also contribute to depression because our body converts foods, such as potatoes, white bread, white rice, to sugar. Bad fats and artificial sweeteners are also a potential risk factor for depression. Whereas a healthy diet dominated by plant-based foods (fruit and vegetables), omega-3 rich oily fish, lean protein, and good fats, such as avocados, can reduce the risk of depression.

Likewise, anxiety, obsessive-compulsive disorder (OCD), attention deficit hyperactivity disorder (ADHD), dementia, bipolar disorder, disrupted sleeping patterns and more are all being linked to our daily nutritional intake.

Society has positioned food as entertainment, and I believe that is a somewhat dangerous approach. Anything that enters our body has an effect. Sometimes good. Sometimes bad. Try to put good nutritional foods and drinks into your body on a daily basis and reposition every else as occasional sidesteps.

Pesticides & Pollutants

In recent years much attention has been focused on the emerging problem with pesticides and pollutants such as plastic and mercury. Links with diseases are beginning to emerge, but we probably won't know the full extent of the damage of our pollutant consumption for many years. These dangerous chemicals have been found in meat, fish and on fruit and vegetables for years. You can start reducing your risk now by embedding a few simple habits. For example, wash your fruit and veg before moving it from your delivery box into your fridge. It's much easier than cleaning each item when you want to eat it. Make it part of the 'putting away' routine. Reduce your meat intake too, so it's an occasional ingredient, not a daily habit. We know that more regularly consuming fish helps us obtain the essential fatty acids we need (omega-3s). However, make sure you reduce your risk of methylmercury exposure and accumulation by eating types of seafood that are lower down the food chain (e.g. salmon, oysters, scallops, sardines). They contain smaller quantities of this toxic substance than the other larger fish who eat them (e.g. marlin, shark, swordfish, some types of tuna). Look up your regional fish to see where they lie on the methylmercury table.

Plastic is another concern when it comes to fish. This fact only hit me two years ago when I stayed in a luxury resort in Malaysia. I arrived in darkness via a speedboat on the island. I felt like James Bond. The following morning, I threw open the shutters of my hut on stilts and was saddened to find an array of plastic bags and flip flops floating past. The resort staff walked the shoreline after every tide to remove the litter that washed in. On my return home, I noticed on the packaging of my prawns that they were from this region. This led me to engage in a lot of research, and now I try to make sure that the fish I eat is from known and clean regions. However, fish is not the only way we consume microplastics. It's also known to be present in our water, sugar, packaged foods and even in the air. Scientists are trying to determine the short-term and long-term impact on our gut microbiome, immune system, brain and body. Aim to make sure your daily nutritional intake is organic fruit and veg from your local farms if you can.

The Next Generation

My mouth is littered with mercury-based tooth fillings from my childhood (we'll explore this in more detail in the Breathing chapter). I am a child of the sugar-fuelled 1970s. Our generation suffered significant tooth decay due to the amounts of sugar-based products that were available to us: lorry loads of easter eggs, candies as free gifts stuck to the front of our favourite comics, the 'tuck shop' at school, the array of TV commercials for various confectionary brands. Sugar was everywhere and seen as a harmless gift. I grew up during the start of the sugar epidemic. This situation continues today, but now children aren't just suffering dental issues; they also suffer weight-related issues. This is a serious situation. We need to wise up, fast.

A healthy, natural diet should be standard practice, but it's not. Almost every establishment I enter features a somewhat compromised and unhealthy selection of food. Why is it so hard to find simple, healthy food in our modern society? Astonishingly, many establishments often don't even recognise that their offering isn't healthy enough. The sugar tax was a helpful step forward but more needs to be done in this direction. Anything that's not aligned with a healthy diet is likely to be seen as tobacco's equivalent when future generations look back at our current era.

My Top Consuming Hacks

I wasn't overweight when I began my experiment, but my weight had been slowly creeping up by about 1lb per year over the past decade. I was undoubtedly on the verge of having to go up a clothing size for the first time in decades. My lifestyle remained pretty active with sport, exercise, gym, but it's a now recognised myth that exercise is linked with weight loss. It actually makes very little impact. Despite my activity this weight-creep was driven mainly by long days commuting to work, grazing on foods grabbed from coffee shops between meetings, and eating and drinking late at night at business events and social gatherings. You can't negate poor eating and drinking habits through exercise and you don't need to be a mathematics genius to calculate that this is how people become obese later in life. It happens slowly and is hard to notice. Even just gaining 1lb per year is enough to result in an obese state by the time you reach your 50s or younger. Most people simply accept it as a normal part of ageing, but that's not true. It's actually driven by our environment and our habits. During the experiment, I made 10 specific but simple changes to my consuming habits, based on various biohacking principles. Within six months, I'd dropped back down to the weight I was in my 20s. I wasn't even trying to intentionally lose weight. It just happened as one of the side-effects of the changes I made to my habits.

Nutrition can often seem really complicated and hard to understand. So, I simplified it. These hacks didn't just fix my waistline; they supercharged almost every aspect of my wellness, from sleeping to focusing on my work. I didn't engage in regular blood glucose testing, although there are many simple testing kits available, even ones that can give you a constant reading. As my weight wasn't at a level of concern, those types of tests didn't seem necessary for my experiment. Here's what I did (in no particular order).

1. I ditched my supermarket habit completely

The lockdown actually did me a favour. I'd been trying to reduce my supermarket visits for many months, but it was the first unexpected Covid lockdown that shut this habit down once and for all. To avoid supermarket visits, I signed up for a great local company that delivers a box of fruit and veg to my door once a week. It looked, smelt and tasted incredible, far better than even the most expensive supermarket produce. The excitement of this delivery each week also greatly exceeded any level of joy that a supermarket shopping experience ever gave me. There was simply no comparison. To shop in a supermarket, I have to drive through town and traffic, park in the car park, push my trolley around endless aisles of food with crowds of other people. Then comes the tedious process of "the checkout". I rarely see anyone I recognise, and there's usually minimal social engagement at the checkout. In contrast, now I have a fabulous weekly stock of delicious food delivered to my door by the wonderful Joseph from Veg Out each Saturday. We have a great chat when he arrives.

This routine also enabled me to focus on the good F words: produce from Fields, Farms and Fishing. I also stayed away from the bad F words: Factory-produced processed food and drink products whose recipes and packaging are intentionally designed to lure my attention and tickle my brain's addictive reward pathways. This weekly delivery automatically resulted in a considerable boost in my fruit and veg intake. I'm not a vegetarian or vegan, but my diet is now heavily dominated by natural plant-based foods and drinks. My consumption of green leafy vegetables has increased most. This has greatly upped my intake of fibre (important for our digestion) and antioxidants (important for clearing daily toxins that build up in our brain). I get everything else, such as toiletries, seafood, cheese and frozen items, during a once-per-month shop at the supermarket or in between at the village shop if necessary. Many people have said to me in recent months that supermarkets form a vital social experience for older adults living alone, but I disagree. There is nothing particularly social about supermarket shopping. No one speaks to you unless you force a conversation. Whereas creating a relationship with your local fruit and veg company is far easier to do. They do speak with you, and you see the same faces who become familiar. I also signed up with my local dairy farmer for a twice-a-week milk delivery, and my neighbourhood baker who delivered my sourdough.

Many people have also said that supermarkets are a much cheaper way to shop, but I disagree. I've spent less since I broke my supermarket habit. How many times have you gone into a supermarket with a list of 10 items, only to leave with many more things than were on your list? These impulse buys don't tend to be cabbages and kale, they're usually unhealthy products that were hard to resist and in hard to miss displays featuring words like DEAL or SPECIAL OFFER. If you compare specific items, then yes, the small local company is probably more expensive than the supermarket. The small companies can't compete with the large chains that buy in mass volumes. However, the saving in your pocket comes from the fact that you're no longer purchasing the additional items you didn't intend to buy before seeing them on the shelf. I've saved a fortune by ditching my habitual "popping to the supermarket" ritual, and I'm much healthier for it.

If you don't have a local fruit and veg delivery company, just set up an online account, so you receive a weekly delivery from your supermarket. Make sure it's dominated by fruit and vegetables. Get your additional treats from your corner shop at the weekend. Stay out of the supermarket environment as much as you can.

I also created my general smart wellness "F'ing Rule of Thumb" for food and drink, and stuck it on my fridge door as a reminder. It's not foolproof because some healthy and unhealthy items can be misclassified and may not be compatible with your gut microbiome. However, I found it a valuable reminder to continue to think carefully about the foods and drinks I put in my body.

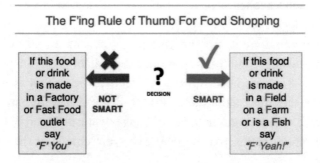

The F'ing Rule of Thumb For Food Shopping

| If this food or drink is made in a Factory or Fast Food outlet say "F' You" | ✖ NOT SMART | ? DECISION | ✓ SMART | If this food or drink is made in a Field on a Farm or is a Fish say "F' Yeah!" |

2. I made a list and repeated it

We've grown to believe that we must eat a wide variety of meals and many different recipes. But our ancestors didn't do that. Even hunter-gatherer societies don't do that. They maintain a staple diet based on the broad range of food they have available in the environment, and they repeat it frequently. I can assure you that by making a simple, repetitive diet your usual routine means the occasional meal in a restaurant is 1,000 times more exciting because it's such a change from the norm. It's a bit like wearing a school (or work) uniform and occasionally having an 'own-clothes day'.

Last year I got into a routine of having an Indian takeaway almost every Friday night. It became a habit, and it became so frequent that eventually, the taste didn't even register any more. I just ate it mindlessly in front of the TV. In contrast, six months after the first lockdown, I decided to venture out and order from my favourite Indian restaurant. It was the most sensational taste I'd experienced for a long time. The level of deliciousness blew my mind, simply because it was so different from my regular fruit- and vegetable-based menus (which were also delicious but in a different way). Less is more. Eating healthily and clean (without flavoured sauces, for example) as a normal practice makes the occasional treats even more enjoyable.

I also tried to make a point of eating more mindfully, taking the time to notice the taste and texture of the food in my mouth. This also significantly enhanced the enjoyment of even the most basic food items. My taste buds seemed to give me more delight than before because I was paying attention to what I was chewing, and because I was eating tastier food direct from farms. I generally ate less but enjoyed it more. I didn't need to add sauces because the food itself became tasty enough. We've become accustomed to eating in front of the television when our brains are engaged in the content being beamed at us, not the food we're consuming. Turn off the TV and give your food more attention. You'll remember how mind-blowingly enjoyable even just a simple tomato is.

3. I made sure I topped up anything lacking

Even though my nutritional intake has improved dramatically due to my increased consumption of fruit, veg and fish this year, I'm probably still lacking in some important nutrients. For example, vitamin D is a fat-soluble vitamin whose main role is to promote calcium absorption, essential for bone, teeth and muscle health. It's also involved in the reduction of inflammation, cell growth, neuromuscular function, glucose metabolism and our immune system. Our bodies make vitamin D from short exposures to the sun, so in the summer I get lots of it from sunlight, but between October and March, I don't. So, I began taking a supplement every day. Because vitamin D is fat-soluble rather than water-soluble, there is a possibility that a tablet may not be absorbed properly by some people's gut. Sprays have been shown to be successful in getting the vitamin into the bloodstream through the lining of our cheek. They also taste nice and minty. Also, I made slight alterations to my wardrobe so that even on colder days I could expose more skin to sunlight by wearing several t-shirt layers that kept my core body warm without the need to cover my arms with a jacket or hoodie. I use sunscreen all year round to protect my skin from harmful ultraviolet rays that penetrate even heavy cloud cover. As well as protecting from cancer, sunscreen helps prevent the development of an uneven skin tone and slows down the damage that ages your skin.

The most complicated aspect of nutrition is that you probably won't notice you're deficient in certain minerals and vitamins unless you get tested.

B vitamins, for instance, are important but hard to maintain sufficiently on a predominantly plant-based diet. They are essential for healthy brain function and are involved in the production of brain chemicals that regulate our mood and emotions, such as serotonin, dopamine and GABA. B vitamins are also important for forming haemoglobin, which is essential for transporting oxygen and carbon dioxide around our bloodstream to our cells. They also play roles in the metabolism of the food we eat and in breaking down fats.

To simplify things, I tried a multi-vitamin by a new company focusing on brain health and function. These guys have combined neuroscience and nutrition to create an all-in-one supplement that's particularly designed for those whose diets are predominantly plant-based. It takes away the uncertainty of whether you're getting sufficient nutrients each day, and it ticks off all the things listed here: omega three essential fatty acids, vitamins A, B1 (thiamine), B2 (riboflavin), B3 (niacin), B5, B6, B12, D3, E, folic acid, zinc, biotin, selenium, chromium, iodine and iron.

To get a more detailed view, I tested my gut microbiome using a test from USA-based firm, Viome. The results were fascinating and helped shape my ongoing nutritional habits. Despite taking supplements of Vitamin D, the test showed I was still low on this during the winter months. I was also low in B12. A few other things cropped up that I hadn't expected, and I'll cover those in later pages.

4. I moved alcohol, sourdough, pastry, chocolate to weekends only

I counted Friday as the weekend, and must confess that during highly stressful weeks, Thursday night sometimes became temporarily classed as 'weekend' too! But limiting these items to weekends meant these days became even more of a meaningful treat than they were already. Due to the nature of our business lives, work can seep into the weekends and sometimes every day can seem very similar. Moving my nutritional treats helped to mark the weekend as different, even if I was working. This move also dramatically reduced my intake of these foods because I wasn't consuming them for four days of the week.

I also switched my milk chocolate habit to a dark chocolate vegan version (and this was before I discovered that my gut was not enjoying cow's milk – see the section about my microbiome test). Milk chocolate delivers no real nutritional value for you. Its sugar-laden recipes and ingredients are designed to trigger the reward pathways in your brain – the ones that can lead to addictive behaviours. Milk chocolate products purposefully try to make you struggle to resist them. In contrast, dark chocolate contains more natural, healthy ingredients – things that are cancelled out by the processed additives and sugars loaded into milk chocolate. Dark chocolate is rich in flavanols which are linked with a range of health benefits for your heart, blood vessels and brain. Choose a high quality, dark chocolate bar that contains a high percentage of cacao (e.g. 70% or higher). It can taste bitter when you first switch from milk chocolate, but once you get used to it, you'll dig it. The bitterness also means that you eat less of it. I put a small square in my mouth and let it melt, sometimes with a coffee. It gives a sufficient hit. I also sometimes eat it with nuts to give it a bit more oomph. Like many people, I used to think I hated dark chocolate, but as with most things, once you've fixed your taste buds and weaned yourself off your sugar addiction, you can enjoy everything more easily. I still enjoy the occasional milk chocolate item, but my dark chocolate purchases dominate.

During lockdown, I signed up with my marvellous neighbour, who has a bakery in his house. He delivered bread to local coffee shops, cafes, restaurants and began delivering to homes during lockdown. A loaf of wholemeal sourdough is delivered to my door every Friday morning. It was the highlight of my week. Not only was it delicious, but it arrived still warm from the oven. There were some days when I sat in the window waiting for it to arrive. I never experienced this level of excitement when I bought my sourdough from the supermarket. Sourdough isn't a health food, but if you can't bear the thought of not having bread in your diet, it's a better choice, as it's believed to have less impact on blood sugar levels. As the name suggests, it's much less sweet than the bread you might be used to, but once you do, you'll probably love it. It's still pretty calorific, though, so don't go mad with portion sizes.

There's more detail about my alcohol intake at point 7 on this list.

5. I bought a filtered coffee machine and embraced decaf

The science of caffeine has received considerable media attention over the years. Sometimes it's heralded as good and sometimes bad. It's been a little confusing. Now, as the evidence builds, some firm facts are becoming apparent. Regular moderate intake of caffeine may indeed hold long-term health benefits. However, I discovered in my research for this book that these benefits can be lost if you regularly consume unfiltered coffee (the type of coffee that most coffee shops serve you and when you use your French press or cafetière). Instead, try to opt for filtered coffee (through filter paper). The paper filtration process removes oils that are believed to be potentially harmful to us. I bought a relatively cheap new filtered coffee machine that I love. You can also use a paper filter holder that sits on top of your mug. I ditched my habitual ordering of lattes and cappuccinos a few years ago, as they were becoming a significant source of calories in my diet. Just switching to americanos with a dash of milk resulted in weight loss when I made that change.

I also axed my habit of having a biscuit with my drink. This reduced the calorie content of this simple habit by 400 calories. I was doing this several times a day when running around London meetings. Now I've taken this change a step further, and instead of asking for an americano (made using their unfiltered espresso machines), I ask for a filter coffee (or sometimes called 'drip' coffee). I embedded other hacks into my coffee routine, and I'll explain those and the brain effects they induce in later chapters.

Alongside my new filter coffee habit, I also occasionally opt for a Bulletproof coffee. You may have heard about this hack already because this drink, and its founder Dave Asprey, have been in the media a lot. Dave is considered the father of the biohacking movement because he first used the term. In brief, a Bulletproof coffee (also known as a butter coffee) is designed to give you an energy boost in the morning and replace your breakfast. It's a high fat, calorific drink containing coffee, butter and oil (MCT oil or coconut oil). It's extremely filling, so it can keep hunger at bay for a long time. It's considered a 'keto' drink.

I'm still trying to drink more water. This is my Achilles heel that I'm still working on. It's the weakest part of my daily consuming habits. I know water is critical for healthy brain and body functioning, but I'm afraid I find it tedious. My water intake is higher than it was at the start of my year-long experiment (also boosted by my increased fruit and veg consumption), but it's still lower than I'd like. To compensate, I make sure that I drink plenty of hot drinks to keep my hydration levels topped up. This has meant that I've had to switch to decaf in the afternoons and evenings so I don't mess up my sleep. Coffee and tea are also good sources of antioxidants, which help neutralise toxic free radicals that build up as waste products in our brain and body. This accumulation eventually damages our cells, particularly our neurons. The imbalance between the production of free radicals and the antioxidants needed to detoxify them is known as oxidative stress. Make sure your diet is filled with antioxidants (available from foods such as green leafy veg, berries and dark chocolate, as well as coffee).

Caffeine is known to interfere with sleep. Adenosine molecules in our brain trigger receptors on neurons that induce sleep. However, caffeine molecules also fit nicely into those adenosine receptors and stay there for several hours. This blocks adenosine from activating those receptors. So, instead of getting sleepy, we continue to feel alert. While this might be useful if you need a boost during a working day, it's not helpful if it then disrupts your sleep patterns. So, after 2pm, I now switch to drinking decaf coffee, decaf tea and green tea. To be honest, I hardly notice the difference between caffeinated and decaffeinated these days because the products are so good. This has enabled me to continue to enjoy hot drinks through the afternoon and evening and maintain my hydration intake, while I keep doing my best to increase pure water consumption.

6. I embraced intermittent fasting

Intermittent fasting isn't as dreadful as it sounds. The word *fast* makes me think immediately of some sort of painful, punishing, difficult and unpleasant challenge. Intermittent fasting isn't like that at all. Intermittent fasting is sometimes also referred to as time-restricted feeding/eating, although I prefer to call it 'time-regulated eating' because the word 'restricted' sounds too negative. It's also referred to as the "16:8".

It's a simple approach to eating and just involved moving my usual meals so they happened within an eight-hour window. For example, I ate breakfast later (around 11am, sometimes midday) and dinner earlier (around 6pm). That left a 16+ hour period when I was not eating anything. The only thing I consumed in the morning was a jug of filtered coffee with a small splash of milk – a drink that isn't likely to break a fast. Tea would have worked too. This fast is pretty easy to achieve because most of it occurs overnight when you're asleep. If you have dinner at 6pm and eat nothing until 10am the next day, you've achieved a 16-hour fast without effort.

Our ancient biology is not designed to eat as frequently and abundantly as we do. Entering a fasted state where our cells have to turn to our fat stores for energy helps maintain a healthy metabolism. They also perform other essential 'housekeeping' tasks during a fasting period. This is known as 'autophagy' and ensure harmful products don't build up in our cells and lead to cell malfunction or cell death. As adults in the western world (who are mostly overeating) it's not necessary for us to eat as soon as we wake up. That myth has developed over time, driven mainly by the advertising campaigns of the sugar loaded breakfast cereal manufacturers. If you frequently pour food into your system (especially carbohydrates), you never reach the stage where you unlock fat stores. Intermittent fasting helped fix the poor eating habits I'd slipped into. It gave me lots more energy, and resulted in a side effect of weight loss over the first four months. Now I use intermittent fasting three-five days per week, and it works great for me. I occasionally use a butter coffee if I wake up hungry (more about that below). However, if I wake up hungry, it's because I've eaten something I shouldn't have the night before. So that's a good reminder to get back on track and pay attention during the evenings.

In the early stages of the experiment, I sometimes used a Bulletproof butter coffee in the morning because I found this more filling. This drink contains grass-fed butter and MCT oil. Grass-fed butter contains good quality fats and helps create a lovely creamy drink that's nicely satisfying and helps keep you fuller for longer. The MCT oil (creator Dave Asprey's version is called Brain Octane C8 MCT Oil) is believed to be more effective than coconut oil in terms of helping your brain and body use fat rather than sugar until you eat again. This helps avoid an energy crash.

A fast helps regulate insulin and hunger hormones. It makes us highly efficient at burning fat for energy as well as glucose. If you're someone who has been abusing your diet regularly with frequent loading of carbohydrates, you may find this new approach difficult.

Mild symptoms known as 'Keto Flu' (more about ketones on following pages) can occur at the beginning, but once you've reset your system, this ketosis stage of a fast can assist with increased mental clarity and energy.

Once I got into the habit of intermittent fasting and not eating until later in the morning or lunchtime, I found I could run fine with just a coffee. This time-regulated eating approach resulted in me eating less in general (particularly late in the evening) because my meals were contained within a smaller timeframe. It worked for me and resulted in weight loss and increased energy that I wasn't even aiming for when I began the experiment. I'm now embedding this as my ongoing normal routine in order to maintain a healthy metabolism.

Fasting has boomed in popularity recently, but it would have been common for our ancestors. Not because they imposed it upon themselves, but because food would have not always been immediately available and within reach. They didn't have refrigerators. They often went for extended periods without eating. Our ancient brain and body circuits respond to food in this way. Continuous eating, snacking and grazing habits, and increased consumption of sugar and carbohydrates, cause chronic insulin releases and screw up our natural systems. Fasting comes in many shapes and sizes and can last for different lengths of time. But it all works on the same principles: once we stop feeding our body, it goes through specific stages. First, it uses the energy that is most readily available – the sugar and carbs we've recently eaten that have been converted to glucose to be taken into cells by insulin for use as energy. Once the available glucose has been used up, your body has to look elsewhere for energy sources – the energy placed in storage cells from previous meals (stored as glycogen in your muscle and liver, and fat in your fat cells). If you want to shift some excess weight, this is an essential stage that you need to enter. It's far easier to enter this stage by focusing on your eating and drinking habits than trying to run off your mistakes on a treadmill every day. We know that exercise has very little impact and is a long and highly inefficient route to fixing a waistline. Instead, focus on fixing your fuel intake mistakes first and foremost. Move your eating and drinking into a smaller consumption window and give your cells regular opportunity to enter a fasted state. For maximum benefits pay attention to your chronotype and align eating and exercising habits with that timeframe. I'm a morning person but you might be a night owl. So test different schedules and stick with whatever works best for you.

Keto, or ketogenic, is a term and a dietary approach that has become common in the biohacking community. It refers to the later stage of fasting when the body switches to burning fat stores, and the liver produces quantities of a chemical – *ketones*. Ketones burn fat for energy. Think of glucose as kindling and fat as logs. The ingredients of Bulletproof coffee are specifically designed to increase ketones. A 'Keto Diet' aims to trigger this ketosis process sooner and maintain it for longer. It does this through an intake of food that is very low in carbohydrates and high in fat. There are various levels of this approach. I would describe my approach as 'casual keto', but at its extreme, some biohackers pay extreme attention to the molecular content of vegetables and associated toxins. I wasn't that serious about it. Intermittent fasting and an occasional casual keto approach worked for me.

You've probably heard the terms' Mediterranean Diet', 'Fasting' and 'Keto' used in recent years but may not have tried them yourself. All three of these eating styles mimic elements of our ancestors' routines. The 'Mediterranean Diet' features mainly fruit, vegetables and fish. It remains the staple diet of many fishing communities in Mediterranean regions – which are also places that have been linked with longer, healthier life expectancy. People in these regions Their alcohol intake is regular but modest and features largely red wine with meals. Extra virgin olive oil is also a daily ingredient in this dietary recipe. There's very little processed foods, and meat is less prevalent than fish and seafood.

As with all these approaches, the best way to achieve good health is to improve your eating habits by consuming moderate amounts of healthy fat, protein and carbohydrates. Achieve this by eating fewer processed foods, carbohydrates, sugar and meat, and have more vegetables, fruit, fish, lean meat, nuts and pulses. Also, reduce your portion sizes to ensure you're not overeating. If you feel stuffed after your meals, your portion sizes are probably way too big. Buy smaller plates and don't eat late at night or too early in the morning. Give your body the time it needs to use up the energy you've consumed the previous day before giving it more. If you filled your car with fuel yesterday but didn't drive it anywhere overnight, you wouldn't return to the fuel station to fill it again in the morning because it still has lots of fuel in its tank. Stop overfilling your tank.

7. I switched from beer and prosecco to red wine

For years, my habitual alcoholic drink order has been prosecco or beer (a lager or a craft ale). As discussed earlier, there is no doubt that too much alcohol is not good for us. However, moderate drinking (e.g. one glass of wine a day) is linked to the Mediterranean diet and other cultural eating habits that suggest it can enhance health. Red wine is known to feature resveratrol, a polyphenol micronutrient that acts as an antioxidant, helping to clear away toxins in our brain and body (although it's only present in small amounts). My drink of choice at home is now red wine, although due to the resulting 'red teeth effect', I don't drink it on a social night out. In those scenarios, I'm trying to switch from beer to spirits, e.g. vodka and tonic. However, the pandemic and the lack of access to social nights in local bars have not allowed me to properly embed this habit. Hopefully, 2021 will see us return to our social lives.

8. I got my gut microbiome tested

As I mentioned earlier, our microbiome is personal to each one of us. It contains a complex combination of microorganisms that are influenced by your diet, environment and lifestyle. They are essential for the efficient absorption of nutrients. It's these bacteria, viruses, yeast, fungi and other microorganisms that do the job of metabolising the foods we eat. For example, it's a little pointless eating spinach if you lack the microbes necessary to convert it into actionable molecules that the body and brain cells can use. The sophistication of microbiome testing now available to consumers is incredible. By sending a small stool sample to the lab, you can get a detailed report with recommendations regarding which foods to focus on, in order to attain maximum wellness benefits. This can give a key insight into how your diet is probably regularly triggering inflammation. This frequent inflammatory response is now being linked with many chronic diseases (not just ones you'd typically associate with diet).

I used a lab that conducts a detailed analysis of your gut microbiome RNA activity. Your DNA is your genetic blueprint. And while our DNA gives us the potential to express genes and produce certain proteins, the process needs RNA to actually happen. Bacteria are single-cell organisms that have their own DNA and RNA and use the same process to express genes. Examining RNA activity shows the actual level of activity of our microbes in our gut.

As I mentioned in a previous section, my results showed a deficiency in Vitamin D and B12. In addition, I discovered a few other surprising revelations. Cow's milk, cheese, tomatoes and grapes were things I consumed daily but were actually irritating my gut lining, even though I had no noticeable symptoms. Apples came out in the test results as one of my most efficient superfoods because my microbiome contains bacteria that can convert this food very effectively without producing blood sugar spikes. So, I increased my intake of apples. I also learnt how to eat apples, because it turns out that I've been doing it all wrong for 50 years. The vast majority of the nutritional content is contained in the core. So, to get maximum benefits from eating apples, we should be eating them from the bottom up, rather than from the outside in. This means the core is hardly noticeable when you eat it. When I reach the pips higher up, I simply spit them out.

My microbiome test highlighted that my inflammation is low (that's good), but my microbial diversity is also low (that's not good). So, I added some probiotics and prebiotics to my daily intake and started eating fermented foods and live bio yogurts. I also now boost my deficient Vitamin D and B12 levels with a more effective supplement. I like the fact that the Viome app allows you to enter foods, to check whether you should be eating them or not. However, the results are hugely detailed and complex, and require an expert with a depth of knowledge to fully explain them. This sort of post-test consultation is a service that Viome surprisingly does not yet offer, so I tracked down a nutritional expert myself to check a few details before making probiotics purchases.

Annoyingly, I got a sudden and unexpected tooth infection just before I was due to take the microbiome test. The pain arrived completely out of the blue, and because we'd just been put into regional lockdown again, I was prescribed antibiotics over the phone. I found this a little irritating, because I don't think I've taken antibiotics in well over a decade, and they're known to alter the microbiome composition and activity. Studies are still trying to determine exactly how long these effects can linger. Antibiotics should only be used as a last resort, and I am not a fan of using them. However, by this point, the toothache was so painful I gladly accepted them.

9. I realised a half-empty fridge is ok

When I used to look in my fridge and see it was half empty, I used to think that I needed to pop to the supermarket. I'd then inevitably end up buying more items than required (see number 1!). This would result in perishable foods from my last shopping trip getting buried under the new items, and then eventually being thrown away because they'd turned bad by the time I re-discovered them. It's a very wasteful shopping habit to eat like this and to ram your fridge so full of food that you just can't see what's in there. When I switched to receiving the box of fresh fruit and veg delivered once a week, this mentally changed. I saw it as my job to eat every single item in that fridge by the time the new box arrived. It also meant it was easier to wipe the shelves clean more regularly. This new approach has made me become much more aware of food waste. Now I hardly throw any food items away. If I start to build up a surplus of any fruit or veg items, I give them to neighbours. This also helps me avoid supermarket environments.

10. I used music

You might wonder how music fits into all this. Here's how I used it to nip my unhealthy consumption habits in the bud.

Since the early 1990s, I've been showing clients how to use positive self-generated cues to help create and maintain good habits and routines. In this case, I used a song to stop myself from automatically reaching for unhealthy food and drink items. Whenever I was tempted to eat, drink or buy something on my NO list, I would sing a song (out loud or in my head). The song I used was *No Limit* by 2 Unlimited. It's a song I know well. The lyrics are pretty straightforward – *"no, no...no, no, no, no...no, no, no, no...no, no there's no limit"* This might seem too simple to be effective, but try it – you might be surprised by the results. Once you've embedded your healthy eating habits, you eventually won't need to use this technique any more. I also used a couple of songs when I was eating or buying healthy items. For example, *I Feel Good* by James Brown and *Reach* by S Club 7. You can just sing them in your head, so no one is aware you're doing it.

In addition to these cue songs, I also used noise-cancelling headphones to block out the supermarket environment as much as possible. I highly recommend this approach for anyone who struggles to avoid making unhealthy purchasing decisions while shopping for food and drink. Remember, supermarkets and the manufacturers of the food and drink they stock use brain science to influence your purchasing decisions. Using headphones is a really effective way of creating a protective bubble around you so you can focus on just quickly finding the things on your list, heading to the checkout, and leaving as soon as possible. I also use specific playlists that make me feel motivated and strong. With some clients, I also encourage them to use guided narration playlists, so they are also listening to a focused talk while they are in the supermarket environment. Try it and let me know how you get on.

DIVE DEEPER

If you found the information in this chapter interesting, I'd encourage you to keep learning about the science of nutrition. There's a ton of great material at your fingertips and some great work being done by exciting academics and practitioners. Here are just a few of the people and sources I've enjoyed reading and following:

Brain Food by Dr Lisa Mosconi
How to Eat Smart and Sharpen Your Mind

The Food Mood Connection by Uma Naidoo, MD
An Indispensable Guide to the Surprising Foods That Fight Depression, Anxiety, ADHD, OCD, Trauma & More

Genius Foods by Max Lugavere with Paul Grewal, MD
Become Smarter, Happier and More Productive While Protecting Your Brain For Life

Drink? by Professor David Nutt
The New Science of Alcohol and Your Health

The XX Brain by Dr Lisa Mosconi
The Ground-breaking Science Empowering Women to Prevent Dementia

The Bulletproof Diet by Dave Asprey

Fast This Way by Dave Asprey

Also, check out some of the great nutritional science courses on the *Coursera* app or website. They're free if you don't want a certification at the end. Just do the course content. It's a great learning platform.

Head to this website below if you want to find out more about fasting and try Dave Asprey's fasting challenge.

www.fastthisway.com

Chapter 4

Breathing

Your breath is a powerful control switch, but you're probably not using it properly

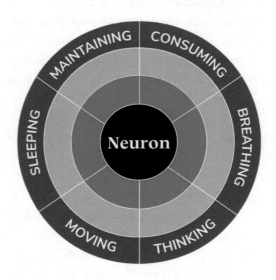

I studied breathing a lot in the 1990s when working as a Sport and Exercise Physiologist, Psychologist and coach. It's an essential measurement for assessing someone's fitness. I also used it extensively when teaching elite athletes how to use breathing techniques to control their anxiety, arousal and heart rate. I've been using it myself and with clients for decades. I thought I knew a lot about breathing, but throughout the research process for this book, I discovered that the science surrounding this natural process had moved forward significantly in recent years.

In addition, there are now also tech devices on the market that can help you supercharge your ability to harness the full power of your breathing.

Let's start with some basic science. Like most people, you might have a basic understanding of the purpose of breathing. You'll know that in order to stay alive, we breathe in oxygen and breathe out carbon dioxide. That's partially true, but the whole truth is a lot more interesting.

The traditional way this topic is taught describes carbon dioxide as the waste product that we need to evict from our body via our lungs so it doesn't poison us. In fact, we need carbon dioxide just as much as we need oxygen, and if you exhale too much carbon dioxide, you soon begin to feel noticeably unwell. We also don't use all of the oxygen we bring into our lungs. Some of it goes back out again when we exhale. Carbon dioxide is actually the trigger that regulates breathing. There are receptors in our brain stem that are sensitive to carbon dioxide in our blood vessels. When they sense the rising level of accumulating CO_2, a signal is sent to the breathing muscles to exhale the excess and take in fresh oxygen. If your receptors are overly sensitive to CO_2, your breathing will be inefficient. The ideal healthy state is to have a greater tolerance to CO_2. This results in breathing less often each minute and means we are very efficient at delivering oxygen to muscles, organs and brain in order to fuel our metabolic process. Remember, if we want our body to use the fuel we eat and drink and avoid gaining weight, we need to provide our cells with oxygen. So, breathing is a vital component of weight loss and weight management. This fact is often overlooked. If you are very efficient at supplying oxygen to your cells, they will be able to burn glucose. You cannot burn glucose without oxygen. In order to fix your waistline, fix your breathing as well as your eating and drinking habits.

By the end of this chapter, you'll see that breathing is a hidden super-tool that can improve bodyweight composition, stress management, sleep, focus and much more. It's the only bodily rhythm that we can consciously control and use to influence other biological systems in our brain and body. This natural act that we do all day and night without thought can be trained. It's highly likely that right now, your breathing technique has fallen into a poor state. Once I started looking at this, I was shocked to find that mine certainly had. I'll show you how I fixed it and the amazing changes that resulted from those adjustments.

My Top Breathing Hacks

1. I used measurements

The first thing I did was to measure my baseline breathing efficiency score. This is something I hadn't done or even thought about for years. I don't have a noticeable breathing problem or any related health issue, so the thought of measuring my breathing ability hadn't occurred to me. Once I measured my breathing technique, however, I was actually quite shocked to see how poor it was.

Here's how you do it. The intention is to measure your level of sensitivity to carbon dioxide by timing how long it takes during a breath-hold to notice the need to breathe. This feeling is known as 'air hunger' as your brain notices the rising CO_2 levels and nudges you to take a breath. Take a few full normal breaths in and out and then at the end of the final exhale, hold your breath and start your timer. Pinching your nose helps ensure that you don't sneak any air in. When you notice the need to breathe, do so. If you're gasping for air during the first, inhale you've held your breath for too long and should do the test again once you've regained normal breathing.

I was amazed to see that my score fell into the fairly poor category. It was just under 20 seconds. I was fascinated and somewhat annoyed by this. I did it several times to make sure, but every reading was the same. I could push it above 20 seconds if I tried harder but then needed a gulp of air afterwards, so it wasn't really a true reflection of my real score. This isn't a test of how long we can hold our breath; it's a test of how long until we notice a need to breathe. Ideally, we should be able to hold our breath for approximately 40 seconds before first noticing the air hunger signal from our brain. Between 20-40 seconds is considered average. Less than 20 seconds is poor and indicates a lack of efficiency in our breathing systems, or possibly high stress or other health issues. It was obvious I needed to pay some attention and work on my breathing technique.

2. I focused on my diaphragm

The first aspect of my breathing technique that I looked at was how I physically drew in breath. I have long known about the importance of using the diaphragm instead of the chest. So I know that I regularly employ diaphragmatic breathing when I am doing relaxation exercises or consciously thinking about breathing during stretches or mindfulness, for example. However, I soon realised that this was not necessarily the way I breathed when my attention was not focused on it. In fact, once I started monitoring it more closely, I often caught myself chest breathing while working at my desk or while out on a walk. Subconsciously it seemed that I was automatically breathing quite shallow and not using my diaphragm as much as I could be. Our diaphragm is a sheet of muscle at the bottom of the rib cage. When it flattens downwards, it creates a change in pressure in that cavity that results in air being drawn in to inflate the lungs. When you are properly using your diaphragm to breathe, you can visibly see your abdomen getting bigger and smaller. Whereas, when you are using your chest muscles, you see your chest rise and expand, sometimes your shoulders too. So, I made a conscious effort to pay frequent attention to my breathing and correct it back to a diaphragmatic technique whenever necessary. The aim was to ensure this became my subconscious automated breathing technique.

3. I used my nose

As well as fixing my mechanical technique, I also paid more attention to how I was taking air into my lungs. I realised with horror that I was a mouth-breather. This really surprised me. However, the more I researched (and watched other people), I learnt that most people seem to have also become mouth breathers. This way of breathing is now known to be the cause of many illnesses, some of which I pointed out in earlier chapters. Our mouth should be closed apart from when we're eating, drinking, laughing, speaking, singing and a few other exceptions.

There are several reasons for this. Firstly, it's important to remember that it's not just oxygen that we suck in when we inhale air. There are other particles in it, some of which are not good for us. Our nose and nasal cavities are designed to filter out these unwanted elements so they don't reach and damage our precious lungs. The hairs and mucus in these areas filter out and trap germs and stop them in their tracks. The nasal passage route is also designed to warm and humidify the air to aid the transition into our bloodstream when it reaches the lungs.

In addition, this channel routes the air so that it gathers nitric oxide from our sinus cavities as it passes through. These molecules play an important role in relaxing our blood vessels and moderating blood pressure. Nitric oxide is also known to be antifungal, antiviral and antibacterial, so breathe through your nose to make the most of this first line of defence against any unwelcome foreign molecules.

All in all, our noses were designed to help us achieve an efficient method of bringing oxygen into our body so we have sufficient fuel. Our mouths were not designed for that purpose, but in recent generations, we appear to have become mouth-breathers. There are thought to be many reasons for this shift. It frequently begins in childhood. Underdeveloped jaws and crooked teeth don't help us form good nasal breathing habits. The resultant mouth breathing makes our dental hygiene even worse because we're inhaling unfiltered germs into our mouth with each breath. It's a negative cycle, but it's one you can fairly easily break once you focus on it. I soon made nasal breathing my norm again and felt much better for it. Endless hours on Zoom during the global pandemic helped me train this habit because it was like sitting in front of a mirror. Every time I noticed that my mouth wasn't closed (except when talking), I made sure I shut it immediately. Before long, my mouth got the message and stayed permanently and comfortably closed except when it was needed. I feel much better for it, and I'm sure my jawline muscle tone has improved too, although this is probably more due to my weight loss than my renewed nasal breathing habit.

4. I breathed low and slow

Throughout our whole life, we're told to take a deep breath when we're stressed and trying to increase calm. That advice is based on the idea that this provides you with more oxygen. In fact, you don't need more oxygen. There is more than enough in every breath, and the body only uses a small proportion of what enters the lungs. The leftover is expelled during your exhale. The trick is to ensure that the available oxygen is accessible by your muscles, organs and brain. To do that, you need to ensure that you have retained sufficient carbon dioxide, not breathe in more oxygen. CO_2 is a critical component in the transportation of oxygen to our cells. Oxygen passes through the lining of our walls and into the blood vessels that surround them. Upon entering the bloodstream, oxygen molecules bind to haemoglobin molecules that are passing by. The oxygen gets carried around the body in our blood vessels by the haemoglobin, like a person in a kayak floating along a river.

CO_2 is acidic. When carbon dioxide amounts rise (because it's continuously being produced by our cells as a waste product of metabolism), the pH level of our blood becomes more acidic. This change in pH level signals to the haemoglobin to release the oxygen so those cells can use it. If you breathe out too much carbon dioxide, your blood pH heads in the other direction and becomes too alkaline as the acidity has dropped. This suggests to your haemoglobin that your cells don't need the oxygen, so it hangs onto it and continues to carry it around the bloodstream. This over-exhalation of carbon dioxide is called over-breathing and causes a range of unpleasant symptoms such as dizziness and shortness of breath. These are commonly associated with feelings of stress and anxiety.

So, deep breaths are to be avoided. The way to improve the efficiency of your oxygen exchange is by breathing lightly and slowly, not powerfully and deeply. A 'low and slow' breathing technique ensures that you don't over-breathe. It enables you to retain sufficient carbon dioxide so that the oxygen that's always in sufficient supply gets released so your cells can access it. Slow down your breathing, use your diaphragm, not your chest, and make sure air is coming in via your nose, not your mouth.

5. I used heart rate variability training

Resting heart rate is a good indicator of health. A high resting heart rate indicates an inefficient cardiovascular system or some sort of underlying problem. As you increase your fitness, your resting heart rate will decrease. This demonstrates that your heart has become stronger and is able to powerfully pump more blood with each beat. It's a muscular organ but, unlike our diaphragm and the skeletal muscles attached to our bones, we cannot consciously squeeze it into action. We can only influence its contractions by increasing the demand put upon it – by increasing our physical movement, for example. Resting heart rate is a biometric indicator that has been an important tool in health for many years. I've used it with my clients for decades because heart rate monitoring devices enabled me to easily measure it before, during and after sessions. By the end of the 1990s, this technology was even built into exercise machines, giving a continuous reading while your hands were on the handlebars. However, I've never in the past paid that much attention to heart rate variability. This wasn't because it wasn't important. It's hugely important, as I'll explain in a moment. The reason I didn't use it was because I couldn't measure it with clients unless we were working in the lab. Today, though, there are numerous tech devices appearing on the market that have opened up this really useful indicator.

Heart rate variability (HRV) is the interval of time between heartbeats (a beat is the little thud we experience when the heart pumps blood out). If you have a resting heart rate of 60 beats per minute, this doesn't mean that your heart is beating exactly once every 60 seconds like a perfect metronome. That figure means your heart contracted 60 times during a minute. The intervals of time between those 60 beats will have varied. You might think that the aim is to reduce the variability and make the heartbeat more consistently. Wrong. In fact, higher variability is better because it is an indicator of the health and function of your autonomic nervous system.

My 12-month experiment focused on my autonomic nervous system in great detail. Many of the hacks and habits I embedded were designed to influence my autonomic nervous system and improve and optimise its function. This branch of our nervous system controls our arousal. It's the system that quickly gets us out of harm's way when we encounter a threat, and that helps us repair our cells, so we're in good condition next time we need to deal with another survival emergency. The autonomic nervous system is connected through its network of nerve fibres to many of our organs. It's divided into two branches, both of which continuously work together to control our healthy functioning. Think of it like a see-saw. On one side is the fight/flight/freeze response. This division – as you'll remember – is called the sympathetic nervous system. The other division is called the parasympathetic nervous system and controls the rest/repair/digest response. As you may expect, it's in our interest to have the rest/repair/digest branch dominating the see-saw most of the time. This helps us enjoy a relaxed life and a healthy body and brain. The balance of the see-saw should only occasionally be switching to our' fight or flight' division when we need a little boost of arousal to get some tasks done, or a huge boost of arousal if we need to engage our muscles and hotfoot it out of a dangerous situation. Unfortunately, our ancient brain frequently confuses the information it receives from the modern environment. If it perceives something as stressful, our fight/flight/freeze division takes over, triggering stress chemicals that over time can be very damaging to the cells in our brain and body. For many people, this can be triggered by traffic, commutes, workload, relationship problems and other things that aren't strictly speaking threats to our survival but act as accidental triggers to your system.

The good news is that once you're aware of this, you can take control of the see-saw because your lungs are connected to it. As we saw above, we have the ability to exert conscious control over our breath because we can choose how we contract our diaphragm muscle.

Here's how it works: the rest/repair/digest division (the parasympathetic arm of the autonomic nervous system) acts as the control. Think of it as a big foot on a brake. Every time we breathe in, that foot releases the brake to allow the fight/flight/freeze division (the sympathetic nervous system) to increase our heart rate a little and move oxygen around the bloodstream. When we breathe out, the foot comes back down on the brake and slows our heart rate down. So, if your autonomic system is working healthily with a strong foot on the brake, your heart rate should go up during an inhale and down during exhale.

This effect involves receptors called baroreceptors that detect changes in pressure in our blood vessels. When our heart rate rises and more blood is forcefully pumped out into the blood vessels, these baroreceptors sense the increase in pressure. They send a signal via our brainstem that tells the brake to re-engage to slow down our heart rate and reduce the pressure. This is a continuous cycle.

The wonderful news is that through training, we can improve the function of this braking system, thereby regulating our response to stress. This has significant effects on our overall wellness. It improves digestion, brain health, and reduces the risk of many chronic diseases that our society sees due to years of having an autonomic nervous system that constantly over-engages our fight/flight/freeze response and its associated stress chemicals (due to a weak brake).

The key player in this game is the vagus nerve. It's one of our cranial nerves that branches out in a huge network and controls most of the parasympathetic wiring (organs that control rest/digest/repair activity). So, you might have heard the term 'vagal tone'. This refers to how well the vagus nerve is functioning. The aim is to improve vagal tone, which basically means strengthening the foot on the brake. I'll explain on the following pages exactly what I did to fix my vagal tone and increase my heart rate variability.

6. I embraced tech for biofeedback

I mentioned earlier that in recent years a number of affordable consumer devices have appeared on the market. This opens up the opportunity to start properly using heart rate variability (HRV) as a key indicator of health and a focus of training. The devices I used for my experiment were the Elite HRV free app, the CorSense HRV monitor (it sends the info from my finger to the Elite HRV app), and the Vagus watch.

Every morning I recorded two readings. They only took a few minutes in total. Firstly, using the finger monitor, I measured my HRV score. This showed me the state of my vagal tone. In other words, how dominant and healthy my parasympathetic brake was and how stressed, or not, I was. Throughout the year, I was fascinated to see

this score improve as I trained it. My baseline soon flew
through the average for my age.

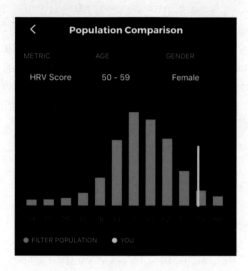

Despite the fact that the fact heart rate variability
decreases with age, I've managed to improve mine to the
point where it's in line with the average score for women
who are decades younger than me, as shown below.

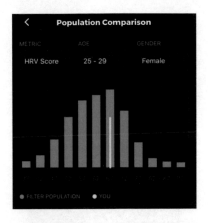

My daily HRV score is now usually in the mid to upper 60s, sometimes in the 70s. Higher heart rate variability indicates a healthy autonomic nervous system. Ideal ranges are 30-100 (measured in milliseconds). You can see my typical daily HRV scores below. The SDNN, RMSSD and HF (high frequency) scores are the important ones as they all demonstrate the health of your autonomic nervous system and the effectiveness of your vagus nerve and the parasympathetic brake. The HF Power score is converted to lnHF (the only time I ever get the opportunity to use my scientific calculator these days), and 4.5 to 7.5 is the average healthy range. Based on the HF measurement of 1712ms below, my lnHF score that day was 7.4, so pretty good. My SDNN and RMSSD scores were also strong in the mid-70s. This indicates low stress, or a high ability to regulate my stress response and keep it under control. In comparison, if you're highly stressed or unwell, these scores would be low.

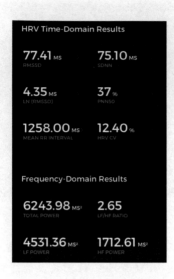

HRV Time-Domain Results

77.41 MS
RMSSD

75.10 MS
SDNN

4.35 MS
LN (RMSSD)

37 %
PNN50

1258.00 MS
MEAN RR INTERVAL

12.40 %
HRV CV

Frequency-Domain Results

6243.98 MS²
TOTAL POWER

2.65
LF/HF RATIO

4531.36 MS²
LF POWER

1712.61 MS²
HF POWER

The chart on the next page shows how my heart rate rises and falls while this heart rate variability measurement is recorded at rest. My general resting heart rate is pretty low. Unlike HRV (which should be high if healthy), a low resting heart rate indicates a healthy cardiovascular system (unless you have some other condition that is causing it)

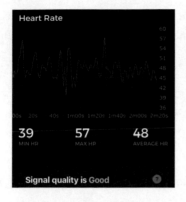
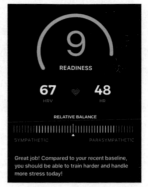

The Elite HRV app also gives you an indication of your autonomic nervous system balance and your "readiness" to deal with stress that day. It was interesting to watch all these scores be negatively impacted by particularly stressful days (or alcohol nights) and then gradually realign again as I got back into my good habits and breathing practices.

In addition to the basic HRV measurement, I also recorded my respiratory sinus arrhythmia (RSA) using the Vagus watch. This may sound alarming, but RSA simply refers to the basic rhythmic cycle of breathing we described earlier whereby heart rate goes up when we inhale and down when we exhale. If this cycle is closely synchronised (whereby our breathing and heart rate remain closely aligned), this indicates a healthy functioning vagus nerve. It cleverly conserves energy by ensuring that blood is pumped to the lungs while they are full of inhaled oxygen. This enables oxygen to efficiently pass into the bloodstream. Otherwise, if the heart was pumping blood past the lungs during an exhale, there would be less oxygen in the lungs available to collect. You can see in the graph below that a healthy vagus nerve does a great job of keeping breathing and heart rate closely synchronised.

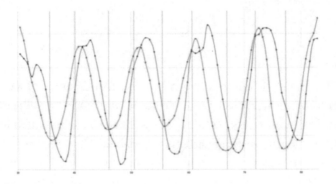

However, the graph on the following page suggests someone who is unwell or highly stressed. Their vagus nerve is clearly not managing to control their heart rate as well as the previous graph. Both breathing and heart rate are much more erratic. The sympathetic nervous system (the fight or flight stress response) appears more dominant than the parasympathetic (vagus nerve) nervous system brake in this example.

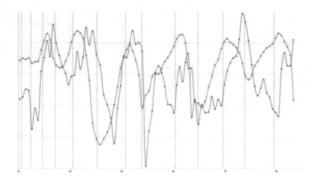

My RSA scores also improved significantly. You can see one of my typical readings in the following graph. The close alignment between my breathing and heart rate is clearly visible. This is good. Interestingly, when I indulged in alcohol, late-night eating, or had poor sleep, this had a clearly negative impact visible on my scores the next morning. It sometimes affected my reading for a few days as my system worked busily to recover from my indulgence. This effect was apparent even if the level of indulgence was relatively small. This really highlighted to me how badly we're damaging our underlying health when we have poor consumption and sleeping habits, especially in relation to alcohol.

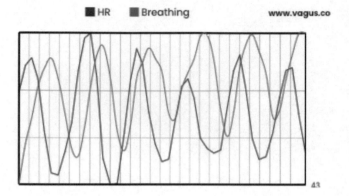

As well as taking daily measurements, I also used these devices to train my parasympathetic brake. This simply involved doing breathing sessions while connected to the devices. It provided me with live feedback showing my HRV and the rate of my breathing to keep me at my resonance frequency rate. Sometimes I did this just for a few minutes, and sometimes I did a full 20-minute session. This was particularly effective when I did it in bed before going to sleep. Learning to slow down my breathing was something I found quite difficult at first, but it eventually became automated and my natural rhythm. Using the devices in this way helped me get in a routine with this training.

I also used tech-powered biofeedback to strengthen the effectiveness of my attentional control. It involved the use of breathing techniques, but I'll explain how I did this using EEG brainwave monitors and virtual reality in the chapter called Thinking.

7. I learnt my resonance frequency

The key aim of my experiment was to find the most efficient practices. I don't like wasting time or money. I want the most efficient techniques and devices that produce the maximum positive effects with the minimum outlay of time, effort and money. Breathing is no exception to this rule, and there are many different breathing techniques if you do a simple search online. For example, box breathing (to maintain a steady, even rhythm) and 4-7-8 breathing with breath-holds (to allow a build-up of carbon dioxide), to name just a few. However, there is a very strong body of scientific research demonstrating that the most effective way to improve heart rate variability, and the associated benefits to blood pressure and emotional mood responses, is by regularly using resonance frequency breathing. As we've seen, there is a synchronisation point when the heart rate and breathing rate aligns. The optimal blood gas exchange is thought to happen when the heart rate increases at the beginning of inhalation and decreases as exhalation begins. This synchronisation occurs when we are breathing at approximately six breaths per minute. However, it's possible to get an even more accurate calculation of this resonance breathing frequency, as I explain below. Breathing at the most precise rate is the most effective in terms of training and improving the vagal tone and stress response. It particularly aligns with the baroreflex element of the parasympathetic response, modulating pressure in the blood vessels.

The resonance range falls within 4.25-6.75 seconds for each inhale and exhale. On average most people's resonance frequency breathing rate is typically between 5.5 seconds and 6 seconds.

To test it, set aside half an hour to do the following measurements:

Breathe for 2 minutes at each of the rates below (making a note of how easy you found the pace – rating of 1 to 5). Wait 2 minutes between each test.

7 (breaths per minute) = 4.3 seconds per inhale/exhale
6.5 bpm = 4.6 seconds per inhale/exhale
6 bpm = 5 seconds per inhale/exhale
5.5 bpm = 5.5 seconds per inhale/exhale
5 bpm = 6 seconds per inhale/exhale

I found the easiest way to do this test was by downloading the free Elite HRV app onto your phone. Under the 'Biofeedback' tab on the app, you can select 'Custom Breathing', and it gives you the sliders to be able to precisely set the inhale and exhale time. Make sure you set the breath-hold times to zero. If you have the CorSense finger sensor (or another sensor compatible with the Elite HRV app), you can also record the average heart rate variability that was measured at each pace. Once you've tried all the different breathing rates, you can see which rate you found the easiest (the one you rated most comfortable) and produced the highest HRV response. This is your personal resonance frequency rate.

If there is a tie between two or more, choose the slowest breathing rate.

Some research advocates a breathing ratio of 4:6 instead of the evenly-timed inhale and exhale ratio I've described above (5:5). This means breathing at six breaths per minute would be a 4 second inhale and 6 second exhale. The longer exhale promotes longer parasympathetic activity and improved training of the vagus nerve activity.

Repeat the test above to measure your 4:6 ratio resonance frequency breathing rate.

7 bpm = 3.4 seconds inhale / 5.2 exhale
6.5 bpm = 3.7 / 5.5
6 bpm = 4 / 6
5.5 bpm = 4.4 / 6.6
5 bpm = 4.8 / 7.2

As your vagal tone and the connections with the baroreceptors strengthen, your resonance frequency may change. So, it's useful to re-check your resonance frequency every three-six months, depending on how much breathing training you're doing. Mine turned out to be 5.5 breaths per minute.

8. I used cold water training

I grew up in the coastal region of West Wales and still live at the beach in South East England. So, sea swimming seems very natural to me. It provides easy opportunities for earthing, which I'll explore in later chapters. It also offers perfect access to cold water. This is true at virtually any time of the year in the UK. The water temperature can rarely be described as warm. Frequent exposure to the cold, and cold water, is something that our ancient ancestors would have experienced. Even in hot climates, the air temperatures drop drastically at night. So, our brains and bodies have evolved with circuits and systems in place to deal with that type of environmental challenge. In our modern world, we have done everything possible to avoid the cold. Warm clothes, central heating systems and steaming hot showers and baths dominate our daily existence.

In the summer months, I often see people at the beach hovering around at the water's edge and making a great commotion about entering the cold water when they decide to take a plunge or even just a little ankle height paddle. I watch them hold their breath or take rapid, deep sharp breaths in between screams as they try and deal with the shock of the temperature change. In comparison, I watch the seasoned wild swimmers all year round enter the water in a much calmer fashion, keeping their breathing controlled and slow. You don't need to have access to the sea, though. You can simply use your shower at home.

As you'll see throughout this book, it's beneficial for us to regularly put our brain and body under a little stress. This prompts our in-built systems to perform their function of keeping us alive. In the previous chapter about consuming, we saw that techniques such as regular intermittent fasting could provide a simple stressor by showing the body a temporarily reduced energy supply. This nudged our body to release stored energy into our bloodstream. Cold water is another easy stressor we can control, which requires our body to respond. This is beneficial for us. In terms of breathing, cold water is an excellent easy stressor because in the early days of attempting this habit, it's often a struggle to maintain control and breathe naturally through the time it takes the body and mind to adjust to the sharp change in temperature. Experts such as Wim Hof' Iceman' have been championing using cold water for boosted health. Using regular cold water and breathing techniques is thought to produce positive effects on metabolic rate, circulation, immune system robustness, alertness and stress responses. It may also stimulate brown fat. In the previous chapter, we talked about the fact that if we overconsume fats, carbohydrates or sugars, they will eventually be converted and stored as fat. There are two types of fat: brown and white. White fat is more dangerous than our brown fat stores and is linked with obesity. Brown fat is activated when we need to generate heat. This is called thermogenesis. Exposure to cold temperature kicks thermogenesis into action. This can have very positive effects on our metabolism because our brown fat cells contain more mitochondria than white fat cells and therefore burn fuel to produce body heat and maintain our core body temperature. As well as being good for maintaining the health of our general metabolic system, it can also lead to weight loss if you are carrying excess white fat stores. There is known to be a 'browning effect', whereby white fat cells can begin to respond to external stressors, such as the cold, by beginning to contain more mitochondria. This effect is stimulated by our sympathetic nervous system, the fight/flight/freeze response when we suddenly find ourselves exposed to environmental stress.

For the purposes of my experiment, I used sea swimming and cold showers as an opportunity to maintain good control over my breathing even when in a taxing situation. The trick is to expose yourself to the water limb by limb, one at a time, while maintaining low and slow breathing. Once you've dipped each arm and leg individually into the cold temperature, the full-body immersion isn't as shocking. Once you've breathed through the first few seconds, it's actually not that challenging. It's even enjoyable. It sends multiple nerve messages from your skin to your brain and kicks the sympathetic nervous system briefly into action, giving you the opportunity to practice pushing down your parasympathetic nervous system brake on it to bring the stress response back under control. This stimulus gives a burst of invigoration as norepinephrine is released in the brain. Try it.

I used cold water training throughout my 12-month experiment simply by ending my usual shower with a burst of cold for a few minutes. However, my daily sea swims ended in November because I have a condition called Raynaud's phenomenon. It's something I first noticed in my teens when outside playing sport in the winter months. This syndrome causes receptors to shut down the blood vessels in my extremities upon the slightest hint of a drop in temperature. They are hypersensitive. Although it's not a dangerous condition if kept under control, it still results in a lack of blood flow to the tissue in my hands and feet. They turn white and then blue and resemble a corpse for quite some time before I manage to eventually get the circulation back to normal again. It's very uncomfortable and rather unsettling. It doesn't happen during my cold showers, so they can continue all year round. But in colder months, the continued drop in temperature once I leave the sea proves too much for my hypersensitive fingers, so I give them a break and stay on dry land with good gloves on.

As well as the benefits described in previous pages, recent research has also started to reveal the possibility that regular exposure to cold immersion during adulthood could potentially provide a level of protection to the brain in old age, reducing the risk of dementia. This effect is not yet fully understood but is thought to relate to a protein produced when we experience cold-shock. This protein is believed to be involved in the formation of new connections between neurons in our brain. This is an ability that becomes impaired in later life and particularly in dementia and Alzheimer's disease.

9. I used physiological sighs

Earlier I said that deep breaths were not something we should be using. However, during the first pandemic lockdown, I heard 'physiological sighs' being mentioned in a talk by Dr Andrew Huberman, Professor of

Neuroscience at Stanford University. I wasn't aware of these sighs before, so I started reading the neurology research. Indeed, I learnt we do regularly sigh even though we don't notice. It's part of our natural breathing process and provides the important function of maintaining the pressure within the hundreds of millions of air sacs in our lungs (the alveoli). The sighs happen every several minutes and re-inflate the sacs to avoid their total collapse due to lowered lung resistance during normal breathing. This process is wired to the vagal nerve. As well as these sighs happening naturally, we can step in and give ourselves a physiological sigh any time we want to engage our vagus nerve and activate the brake, for example, at moments where we are feeling stressed or anxious. To initiate a physiological sigh, take a normal breath in, but then quickly breathe in some more. This pops open the air sacs to their maximum capacity, and the stretch receptors trigger an intense activation of the vagus nerve. This deactivates our stress response and re-engages the brake. Then, breathe out gently and slowly because, as I mentioned earlier, this keeps the vagus nerve engaged during exhalation. This physiological sigh is a very useful tool and something I actually used quite a lot during the stress of the first lockdown when the pandemic hit. Note that this sigh is different from the emotional sighs that you might do consciously or subconsciously during periods of frustration or distress. Those often have noticeably fast, forceful exhales and aren't delivering the positive impact I describe above.

10. I used music

As usual, I used music frequently as part of my breathing training. It's the perfect tool because it's rhythmic. Once I had determined the breathing rate I needed to maintain, I was able to find songs that matched the tempo. This enabled me to regulate the pace of inhalations and exhalations without having to stare at a stopwatch or screen. Chilled, relaxing songs also helped me get into the right mindset for slowing down my heart rate, and breathing and engaging the rest/repair/digest parasympathetic brake. Songs that we know well are so deeply ingrained in our memory that we can even reproduce them in our mind with quite consistent accuracy. This means that even when I just sing them in my head, I can be reassured that my breathing is approximately keeping the right rate. Being able to call upon a song in your mind like that means this activity can be done anywhere at any time. For that reason, it's a very versatile tool because you don't need to have the actual music with you. Prior to the pandemic, there were many times early in my experiment that I called upon my go-to song cue to regulate my breathing during unpleasant rush-hour crushes on the London Underground. Enabling me to breathe through the horror and anxiety of it, ensured my vagus nerve kept that parasympathetic brake firmly engaged to keep my fight/flight/freeze stress response under control. One of my songs of choice in this scenario is Natalie Merchant's *San Andreas Fault*. Find songs that work for you. It enables me to inhale over 6 seconds and exhale over 6 seconds, which is approximately my resonance frequency rate. Also, I know that sometimes when I'm in a stressful situation, I may be reproducing the song in my mind at a slightly higher tempo. However, because the actual rate is 6 seconds, then I know that even if I'm accidentally speeding the song up a little, I'm still going to be within a decent tempo for regulating breathing. Whereas, if I was using a song that had a tempo that maintained a rate of 4 seconds for inhaling and 4 seconds for exhaling, I would likely not be getting a relaxation effect if I accidentally sped that up when singing in my head. So, choose a song at the lower end of your repertoire if you're in a stressful environment and don't have your headphones with you.

Obviously, using music is straightforward if you're using the 5:5 breathing ratio because the equal timing of your inhalation and exhalation synchronises with the standard tempo of songs. However, if you're using the 4:6 ratio breathing, it's much harder to align this with songs unless you're using music that has a tempo that aligns with this uneven ratio.

Incidentally, humming a song at a low pitch has been shown in some cases to increase the production of nitric oxide in the paranasal cavities. I tried this but decided I didn't need it badly enough to make it part of my daily routine. However, if I developed a condition that would be improved by an increase in nitric oxide levels, I would definitely add this simple technique into my day.

DIVE DEEPER

Here are some of the books related to breathwork that I absolutely loved. If you want to continue to build your knowledge and dig further into the science of breathing, here's some recommended reading.

The Oxygen Advantage by Patrick McKeown

Just Breathe by Dan Brule

Breath by James Nestor

The Wim Hof Method by Wim Hof

Jaws: The story of a hidden epidemic by Kahn and Ehrlich

Biofeedback and Mindfulness In Everyday Life by Inna Khazan, PhD

Chapter 5

Thinking

We can choose how our brain perceives and responds to the information it receives from the outside world. Your perception and your thoughts mould your reality

Mental health care will cost the world $16 trillion by 2030 (Lancet Commission)

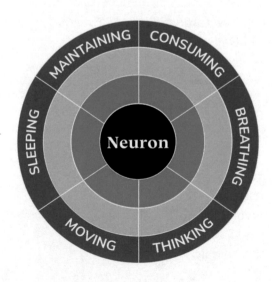

When I first became a coach, I learnt that we have significant control over how we perceive situations in which we find ourselves. We can influence this process before the event, in the moment, and continue to do so after it's happened. As humans, we can look forward to, or worry about, things that haven't yet happened; and positively celebrate, or negatively ruminate over, something that happened in our past. There is a significant variation in how people respond to events. Two people experiencing the same situation can react and be affected by it in very different ways. Someone who is very much in control of how their brain perceives stimuli and understands the underlying evolutionary biological processes is more likely to maintain control, even in highly stressful situations. I showed young British athletes how to use music, breathing and visualisation as powerful hacks to quickly achieve the desired mindset such as calm, focus and achievement. This allowed them to draw on these tools whenever they needed to relax in a tense moment of competition or maintain motivation during long gruelling training periods. I believe everyone should be taught these skills. They can be life-changing. In this chapter, I will show you how I strengthened my ability to control how I perceive my world, thereby boosting my resilience, performance and wellness.

Let's start by looking at the mechanics of this process and how it relates to wellness. At its most basic level, the process involves our brain receiving information from the outside world via all our available senses. I use the word 'available' because perhaps in some situations, information isn't available via all routes. For example, if your eyes are closed, you're not receiving external visual information, or if you have earplugs in your ears or have a hearing impairment, you're not receiving all external auditory input. Also, not all frequencies are available to us. For instance, my dogs can detect sounds and scents that are not available to my human senses. The world as we know it is confined to the way our evolutionary brain perceives it. In the very distant future, who knows how our brain will continue to develop to detect an even greater range of frequencies and energies. Perhaps we'll invent technology that can help our brain to sense additional information in our surrounding environment. The whole concept is fascinating.

Our world is simply a bunch of vibrating atoms when you zoom down to its tiniest particles. They are the building blocks of everything in our world. Even the air we breathe is composed of atoms that have joined together. These are known as molecules. Molecules that bind together are known as compounds. A molecule of oxygen, for instance, is made of two oxygen atoms, which is why it's called O_2. Water is made of two hydrogen atoms and one oxygen atom – H_2O. So, we're surrounded by atoms. Even our body is made of atoms clumped together in different ways. Atoms are the building blocks of everything in our world. However, we don't need to become particle physicists to boost our wellness. All we need to remember is that the physical matter around us is made of tiny vibrating atoms. Light is made of tiny particles called photons. Sound is the vibration of air molecules that have been triggered by the vibration of an object. All of these particles have meaning to us because we place significance on them. We can choose what meaning to put on this sensory information we receive from the outside world.

The available information reaches our brain via our senses and the peripheral and central nervous system fibres (think of it like train tracks heading to the central hub station). The usual electrical and chemical responses are triggered as action potentials travel along neurons. These action potentials activate relevant regions of the brain and body to initiate whatever response is deemed to be required based on the analysis of the sensory information received (and compared with memories of similar past experiences). For instance, if an external environment is perceived as threatening, a level of stress response will be initiated, causing the heart rate and breathing to increase, and more blood to be diverted to our muscles so that we can run for our life. The thalamus and other structures in our limbic region play a vital role in this process of relaying and responding to all this information. Our memories and past experiences also greatly influence our perception. Importantly, all this is happening continuously without us being consciously aware of it.

General wellness is often thought of in terms of three aspects: health, wealth and happiness. If you have all three of these in abundance, there should be a lack of stress in your life. If one of these is off, then it can also negatively impact the other two. People can experience these three aspects in contrasting ways. For instance, two people with similar lives can perceive their level of happiness differently. Assuming there are no underlying neurological impairments, this judgement is being made because of how we perceive our external environment and the prior experiences we've had. Similarly, two people with the same amount of money in their bank account can consider themselves either wealthy or not. It depends on their level of financial outgoings and their expected level of wealth achievement. The direction of travel of a bank balance can induce feelings of extreme stress. Someone who has several children at an expensive school and a massive house with a significant mortgage can soon find their stress response is triggered if they see their funds dwindling. The pressure on them intensifies to reverse this situation and find income solutions to reverse the flow before life changes have to be made (e.g. selling the house or pulling the kids out of school). The negative impact of stress can also reduce the likelihood that a positive outcome will happen. It's a problematic negative cycle.

Money has become a core influencer of wellness because so much of our existence is now dictated by it. Yet, for most of us, myself included, it's not something we're taught to seek in large amounts. Some of us have very limiting beliefs regarding how much money we will earn in a lifetime. This is primarily influenced by your upbringing and the level of wealth your ancestors achieved. As part of my experiment, I engaged in a general wheel-of-life evaluation and was interested to find that finance was actually the aspect that leapt off the page as the rustiest spoke in my wellness wheel. The nature of my work is mostly project-based. It's often a slightly precarious existence. I used to tell myself that I enjoyed the thrill of it because there's always a buzz of brain chemicals when you finally land a new, exciting, and well-paid project. However, when I sat down to complete a detailed evaluation, it became clear on paper that this was not an ideal situation and certainly not a route to lifelong wellness.

There's no escaping the fact that modern humans need to build stable income, wealth and financial freedom. Freedom is the key word. This freedom removes many stressors that can chip away at your underlying wellness without you noticing. It's a constant little trigger of your stress response. There are four ways to tackle this, and you need to address them all.

First: you can learn to strengthen your autonomic system so that these constant external stressors have less effect on your biology because your parasympathetic brake can maintain control.

Second: you can regain control of how you consciously perceive stressors, so they become less likely to trigger a stress response.

Third: you can remove the subconscious limiting beliefs that exist in your daily existence without you noticing them.

Fourth: you can remove the financial stressor, either by reducing your outgoings or increasing your income.

I found it fascinating that I had such limiting beliefs regarding the level of my financial value. We're often taught that chasing money and wealth signifies greed – 'a negative thing'. That's simply not true. Wealth enables you to achieve greater wellness for yourself, your family and your friends. It allows you to do good things for others as well as yourself. I've spent in the region of £100,000 on my education and building up my expertise over the past 25 years. Yet it's clear from my evaluation that I'm not extracting the full potential value from my knowledge. As part of my experiment, I decided that I needed to change my approach to wealth, cast off limiting beliefs about finance, and boost my income. I also aligned my financial goals with my purpose of wanting to help people enjoy a lifetime of good health. You'll see how I did this later. Bear in mind that it was wealth that popped out as my weakest link. This is why I targeted it in my experiment. However, all these elements are also highly related. You may find that health or happiness stand out in your life, not wealth. When I'm experiencing financial stress, even if just at a small or unnoticeable level, this can impact my perception of overall happiness, which can eventually impair my physiological wellness due to the chronic engagement of my stress response and the resulting chemicals and inflammation. It will impair my sleep quality, the way I engage with those around me, my motivation levels, and so on. If you find that health or happiness is the rusty spoke that needs attention, the following pages equally apply to you. These hacks are designed to give you greater control over how you perceive your world so you can make changes and improve your happiness, health and wealth.

As humans, we have a unique ability to take a step back and use our knowledge to consciously change our brain. This is an incredible power. The ancient development of the prefrontal cortex region of our brain's frontal lobe has given us this gift to be able to consider what we think. We're able to assess situations, critically analyse, plan, make decisions, evaluate our performance. We were much better at these things than our Neanderthal relatives. They had larger brains than us, but that was because the occipital lobe at the rear of their head was larger than ours, not their frontal lobe. The occipital region is responsible for processing visual information from our eyes. We had the larger, more developed prefrontal cortex region. So, they could probably see better than us but could not think, plan and analyse as well as homo sapiens could. This awareness is known as metacognition, and it's enabled us to dominate other creatures and take over the planet. It's also your steering wheel to lifelong wellness and a healthy, wealthy and happy life. You can use knowledge, assess a situation and make changes that influence the outcome. This book gives you knowledge in the form of fundamental science tips, and the hacks are changes you can embed in your life to influence the outcome. You can change how you perceive things and how you respond to them. At first, this needs to happen consciously because you may need to break existing, habitual responses that you've been doing for so long you've engrained them subconsciously. Remember, the brain aims to conserve energy whenever possible. It's a gas-guzzling engine that makes up just 2-3% of your body's weight but consumes a whopping 20% of your daily energy burn. In order to use less fuel, it's cleverly evolved to choose routine responses because they can be carried out automatically, without thought, requiring less neuron activity and, therefore, less fuel. *It's vital to remember this*. This ability to run automated 'programs' is our blessing and our curse. You may be running subconscious programs that have bugs in them due to previous experiences or beliefs. Fortunately, once you've identified them, it's possible to update, replace or re-program them using your unique human superpower of metacognition.

Reframing how you decode and respond to information is a powerful advantage. Having a greater awareness of what's happening helps you to control your response. This process can be improved through training. It can help reposition chronic stressors that you encounter in your daily life. It can help cast off limiting beliefs, fear of failure, inability to focus, or help you be inspired by your everyday life. Of course, beliefs and responses related to significant past trauma or phobia require more work. For this experiment, I simply aimed to enhance my ability to control my brain state and thoughts in order to boost focus, happiness and get rid of a few limiting belief shadows. Stress and anxiety, even at low and almost unnoticeable levels, can mess with attention, memory and your ability to stay in control of decisions and thoughts. Science confirms that our emotions and our cognitive function are linked. Our feelings are rapid survival-based responses, such as fear. When those emotional states continue for more extended periods, we call them moods, such as 'happy' or 'sad'. The limbic system region of our brain and our brainstem are significant players in these instinctive emotional reactions. The good news is, we are able to step in and exert a level of control. The changes I made to my daily life significantly influenced and improved my control over how I perceive past, current and future experiences. Here are my top 10 tips. My aim was to supercharge my mindset and my ability to focus and learn, maintain control over stress and emotions, and move rapidly and intently towards goals.

My Top Perceiving Hacks

1. I fixed my environment and created a routine

Once you realise that the brain is continuously being influenced by the information it's receiving, without you being consciously aware of most of it, it makes total sense to make sure your external environment doesn't contain negative features. Remove as much negative sensory 'noise' from your surroundings as you can. I did a simple analysis of my area, and a few problems became glaringly apparent. I addressed each sensory input as best I could.

i. Vision

This one was easy. It was evident that there's a lot of clutter around me— both inside my house and in my garden. So, I took action to reduce the amount of visual chaos I was surrounded by. I finally got around to paying someone to come and fit a loft ladder, so I could move all the boxes from the room I use as a home office area. This room had become a dumping ground. I took this one step further and rented an office, so none of it needs to be in my home at all. I also tried to embed a 'put it away now' response. This is not something that comes naturally to me. My habitual reaction is 'put it away later' but 'later' never usually comes. All those items lying around just continue to tell your brain 'INCOMPLETE'. I tried to get disciplined about looking at my surroundings and removing everything that didn't need to be there. I particularly focused on my bedroom, and I'll explain that in greater detail in the chapter about sleep. I also tried to maintain this approach for my desk. Every day, as part of my routine, I tried to find five things to put away. I also took into consideration things that weren't sending my neurons the appropriate message. For example, I realised that some of my coffee mugs had slogans such as "I'd rather be walking the dog" or "Keep Calm and Have A Cupcake". These are fun concepts, but they're not exactly messages aligned with the things I was trying to achieve. So I replaced them with mugs featuring images or slogans such as "Today I Can Do Anything". Remember that your brain notices these things even if it decides to not make you consciously aware of them. Choose your surroundings carefully.

In addition, I bought some new dimmer lights, and I'll explain that in more detail in the sleep chapter.

ii. Sound

This one was also pretty easy. I used music extensively to create an influential sound environment for my brain. It became clear that I wasn't extracting the maximum value from sound in my home environment. I own a lot of audio equipment, but most of it isn't set up properly, so it's not used. I addressed all that, and now I can play soundscapes in most used rooms at the touch of a button.

iii. Touch

I decided which pieces of furniture I found brought me joy and the ones I did not. I reshuffled them so the pleasing items were in positions where I could use them more regularly, and removed things that I didn't like or want. I also bought some things to enhance this impact — for example, a new weighted blanket for my bed and a new cushion for my chair.

iv. Smell

This one's an interesting one because sometimes you don't notice smells that you're always surrounded by. For instance, as a dog owner, I don't notice the doggy aroma that visitors probably get hit with when they arrive through my door. I did begin to light candles much more frequently and made that part of my routine. I also started really paying attention to my coffee in the morning, enjoying the aroma of the bean grinding process and savouring the smell of the freshly-brewed coffee in the mug when taking my first sip. I also made a point of opening windows more often to ensure a regular cycle of fresh air through the areas I was working in.

As well as fixing my environment, I created a routine. This routine is detailed in Part Two of this book. Some of the most critical habits in this routine were the morning ones. They were specifically designed to boost levels of chemicals that made me feel positive, happy and energised. This sense of how we feel is known as affect. Affect is experienced through feelings of arousal (are you calm or highly agitated) and valence (are the feelings you're experiencing pleasant or unpleasant). Many of the hacks in this book are intended to help ensure we're experiencing optimal levels of arousal – calm when necessary and energised and enthused when necessary – and valence – experiencing positively pleasant feelings.

2. I kept the chimp in check

This is probably one of the most important points of this entire book. You'll remember I've mentioned the limbic region of the brain several times already. This collection of brain circuits operates and is driven by survival instincts, the law of the jungle. It's very, very powerful. One of my favourite books is *The Chimp Paradox* by Professor Steve Peters. He calls our limbic centre "the chimp". Once you learn how the chimp thinks and behaves in response to environments and experiences, you will take a giant leap forward in being able to control your emotional reactions and how you enjoy life.

The chimp is continually pulling and pushing levers which can wreak havoc with internal physiology and wellness. The chimp is impulsive and lacks control. It is powerful, but we have the ability to use our frontal lobe regions to step in and influence its behaviour. The chimp is why your previous attempts at diets and exercise fads have not given you lifelong wellness or a fabulous waistline. The chimp makes decisions based on survival. If you don't go to the gym today, will you die? Your chimp assesses the situation and thinks probably not. The chimp says yes when someone asks you if you want another beer or a cake with your coffee. So, the question is: 'do you want your chimp to be dictating your life, or do you want to keep it in check and use your human power to assess whether a certain response or action is required or not?' The first step in that journey is to understand that this chimp (your limbic system) exists and it's operating on ancient evolutionary rules based on survival decisions. The second step is to learn how to take its power away. This can be done through various training practices I describe below, and through techniques you can do in the moment, such as distractions or cues. For instance, I mentioned in the previous chapter that I sang the "There's No Limit" song in my head when confronted with a food item I knew I should avoid. Switching your thoughts to something else can help stop or alter the chimp's automated activity and the consequent effects of its actions.

3. I strengthened my control switch

As well as keeping the chimp in check to avoid unwanted and misinformed, emotionally-driven stress responses, I also realised that I needed to give my brain a little help in maintaining focus. Our salience network is a collection of brain circuits that act as an attentional switch. It flicks between two networks known as our central executive network and default network mode. These networks operate regions of neurons that either help us to maintain focused attention on something (e.g. a task that needs our full conscious attention and awareness) or a mind-wandering mode if our full attention is not required. Both of these modes are necessary for healthy function, but sometimes mind-wandering mode switches on at inconvenient times and interrupts our concentration. To gain better control over this salience network and my ability to switch between brain states, I embedded some training practices.

Most of this practice happened with my eyes closed. I used self-hypnosis and guided meditation to become much more adept at entering different mind states and moving between them. The enhanced ability to drift into a trance-like state by slowing brainwaves and thoughts definitely improves with effort. There are many different ways of doing this and a wide variety of self-hypnosis and meditation guided videos online. Try some and find the ones you like best and that work for you. At first, you'll find it difficult to stop the chaos of distractions crashing around in your mind. The more you work at it, the easier it becomes to silence that internal chatter and maintain focus. I started teaching self-hypnosis, guided breathing and meditation to students in the 1990s as an elite sport psychology technique. However, I'd fallen out of the habit of doing it in my own life. So, I made sure it became part of my new daily routine. I tried to do it first thing in the morning while taking my HRV, RSA and sleep readings. Also, in bed at night before drifting off to sleep. Additionally, I tried to drop in a little bit of mindfulness during the day with my eyes open or shut. This was to train my brain to stop leaping around and maintain focus.

I also introduced some panoramic gaze practice into my working day whenever the workload began to feel a little overwhelming. This is a technique I discovered from Dr Andrew Huberman, Neuroscience Professor at Stanford University.

Human vision is wired to our autonomic nervous system fight/flight/freeze response. This is obvious when you think about it because, to survive, you need to rapidly absorb visual information to determine where the threat to your survival lies and how to avoid it. When you focus, it's to increase the amount of visual information you can gather on the target. In contrast, when you're in a non-threatening environment, your visual focus is more relaxed and able to gather information from the wider surroundings. By consciously switching to a comfortable, soft panoramic gaze, you're helping to disengage the sympathetic nervous system and re-engage the rest/digest/repair parasympathetic nervous system mode. To achieve a panoramic gaze, simply look straight ahead but take in all the visual field to your left and right at the same time. I believe this peripheral vision training is a potent tool because it can be done so easily and quickly. I haven't managed to find much detail in the scientific literature about this effect, but it stands to reason that prolonged staring at screens results in spending very little time in a relaxed panoramic gaze mode.

Interestingly, Andrew Huberman also uses the opposite visual technique when aiming to do some focused work. He stares intently at a mark on his wall in the distance before starting work on the task. This is thought to help engage a low level of sympathetic arousal, resulting in an increase in delivery of acetylcholine in the prefrontal cortex. As you read in chapter 2, acetylcholine is an important chemical component in focus and learning.

4. I used tech to improve my practices

As with my breathing practice, I used tech devices to give me information that helped improve my training success. Using heart rate and heart rate variability monitoring for live or post-training biofeedback helped me check the effects of my thinking and breathing activities on my brain and autonomic nervous system activity. I also tried virtual reality (VR) tools and found some great breathwork exercises that involved me controlling the movement of waves on a beautiful beach and flowers in a scenic field using my inhalations and exhalations. However, I found that the temperature of the headset became warm during the practice sessions. By the end, I would emerge with a hot, red face. I also used devices such as the Muse headband to monitor brainwave activity to help me focus on slowing down my thoughts and boost focus. This is helpful in basic early-stage training when you're learning how your thoughts are represented through increases in electrical activity. However, I found the constant audio feedback too distracting when I began to train for a drift into slower brain states, from beta brainwaves down to alpha and theta. For those sessions, I used guided self-hypnosis or meditation recordings rather than the audio from the headband. Those sessions proved to give me a much clearer connection with my subconscious. This was something I hadn't engaged with regularly for many years. Most of us aren't maximising the potential of our brain because we have a very superficial understanding of and engagement with it. The power of our subconscious mind (the things that are happening without our conscious awareness) is hugely untapped and uncontrolled by most people. The medical profession now recognises how closely our subconscious processes dictate our wellness. I'm having a lot of fun submerging myself deep in these areas of my mind and programming them with things that I want to achieve (health, wealth and happiness), experience and enjoy.

5. I used gratitude to boost brain plasticity

I must confess that although I consider myself a grateful person, and certainly try not to take things and people in my life for granted, I'd never before engaged in gratitude practice. It's highly connected to the techniques I described above in terms of its link with our emotions, our subconscious mind, and beliefs. However, my interest was piqued even further when I read about the physiological effects of gratitude that are so apparent they can be visibly seen on a brain scan. The brains of monks who engage in regular meditation on gratitude have a good density of neurons in regions of their brain that are linked with attention. They have a high level of control over their ability to switch between brain states. It also helps combat the brain's natural decline of neurons as we age. Monks have been seen to display much lower levels of biological ageing in their brain tissue due to their meditation routines. As well as adding gratitude to my regular mediation and self-hypnosis practices, I embarked on a daily little gratitude habit. Every morning while my coffee brews, I head into the lounge and spend a little while telling my dog about all the things I'm grateful for. I stroke him gently while I'm telling him all this. He absolutely loves it, and so do I. In fact, if he now hears the coffee machine start to brew and I haven't yet arrived in the lounge, he comes to get me. Sweet. If you don't have a dog, just write your gratitude in a journal. It doesn't matter if you're grateful for the same things every day. I am. I also discovered that many financially successful people include their gratitude for financial freedom in their daily practice and began doing that even before they had economic freedom. I started doing this too. I specifically stated every day that I'm thankful that money comes frequently and easily. It was fascinating to see how this one actually began to change and increase my income streams. I was fascinated by this, and I'll explain it in more detail later.

6. I smiled a lot and worked less

I smile quite a lot. I have a good sense of humour and spend time with people who are similar. Laughing and smiling is usually a natural part of my day. However, I realised that as soon as lockdown happened, my smiling decreased. This was due to two reasons. Firstly, we were in a pandemic, and that's not really an experience that induces smiling. Secondly, I was suddenly living alone because care duties separated our family geographically. I was smiling less because I wasn't socially engaging with other people as regularly. So, I made a point of smiling and frequently talking with my dog, on Zoom meetings, and when out on my daily walk seeing other people, even if just from a distance. Smiling sends important signals to your brain. It represents a situation that's relaxed, happy and enjoyable. This sends vital information to your chimp and boosts brain chemicals that make you feel good. I've also read research suggesting that holding a pencil in your mouth can trigger this brain response because it engages facial muscles responsible for smiling. However, I didn't need to go to those lengths. I organised weekly 15-minute dance sessions and singalongs on Zoom for my friends and colleagues. These sessions were a fun way of goofing around in what were otherwise relatively quiet days for me at home on my own with Charlie pup.

I also added a smile game to my daily walks. Every day I tried to pinpoint five things that I saw during my walk that made me smile - for example, a flower, a sunset, a person's funny walk, a cute dog. It doesn't really matter what it is. This also helped me stay in the present and appreciate my surroundings, rather than drift into mind-wandering mode (although sometimes I decided to do that as well). Smiling and laughing are an essential aspect of wellness. It's also worthwhile evaluating your working hours. Often we spend far too much time at our computer. Usually, it's because we don't want to be judged by employers, clients or colleagues as 'slacking'. In reality, most of the time you spend at your computer is unnecessary. It tends to induce frowning, not smiling, and it's pouring blue light into your eyes, which is not something you want after sunset. I arranged my day so that I completed focused work in the morning and a few scattered meetings in the afternoon. I tried to not work at all after 6pm. I began working much shorter hours but achieving much more.

7. I re-discovered my strong sense of purpose

When I first graduated as a sport and exercise scientist aged 23, I had a very strong sense of purpose. My undergraduate degree fired me up and inspired me to want to go out and help the world get healthier. I maintained that sense of purpose throughout the 1990s, teaching thousands of clients and students how to improve their health and how to teach others to do the same. However, after a decade, I began to get a little disillusioned. It was clear that the fitness sector wasn't going to create a healthy population. I watched endless streams of people sign up to join gyms and start a programme, but very few made the lifelong changes to their lifestyle necessary to fix their health. Over the years, I watched them age poorly. Even using psychological tools didn't succeed because the things we were asking them to do didn't align with the priorities of their inner chimp. It was too difficult for them to fight the chimp and force themselves to stick with fitness routines that were not strictly speaking necessary to survival at that moment. The same was true of diets. They stressed the chimp in the wrong ways. However, this model was hugely successful financially because most people have a burning desire to be healthy. There is always a vast target group of potential customers. The health club division I developed for a relatively small family-owned hotel chain grew to become a highly successful part of its business. It helped drive expansion as they bought more hotels. In every new location, there was a population of people keen to improve their health and subscribe to become a member of the hotel's private health club. The hotel group eventually sold for £180 million, instantly transforming the family and board of directors into multi-millionaires. It was fascinating to be part of that journey.

I left the sports, health and fitness world and, after a brief post-MBA encounter with commercial finance and investment banking, moved into the experiential marketing and events sphere. I started getting paid to help corporate clients use the same behavioural science principles I'd used with athletes and health clubs, to build experiences that engaged their customers. In other words: fun and enjoyable music-filled social environments and events. This was fun but didn't really give me a sense of purpose. It was my doctorate that brought me back around to a sense of purpose. Initially, my PhD research was spurred by the visible lifelong effects of music people remember from youth. I spent nine years researching this topic and examining how and why these experiences become so deeply embedded in our memory. I began to realise these lifelong attachments could also be purposely be used to produce specific effects. For instance, using music memories can engage a person who is lost in the later stages of dementia. This phenomenon brought me back to the field of wellness and inspired a sense of purpose. It was gratifying working with dementia organisations to embed music in care practices, but I saw an even greater need to teach people how to look after their brain throughout life, so the risk of their neurons declining towards dementia was greatly reduced. That's what formed the seed for my experiment, this book, and the subsequent training courses. I once again have a sense of purpose and a drive to achieve these goals. They will not only enable me to 'do good' by helping people improve their wellness, but also will stabilise my own health, wealth and happiness.

8. I set structured goals

It won't surprise you to learn that as someone whose journey began in the sports sector, I'm a big fan of goals. I've been using them in client work and in my own life for almost 30 years. I can guarantee that goal-setting is one of the most effective hacks you can use to achieve lifelong wellness.

First, though, you need to know what the goal should be. Experience has taught me to make them as simple to reach and as exciting as possible. 'Losing weight' isn't exciting or straightforward. It's a statement that's impossible to measure. 'Losing 10lbs and then buying myself a new (insert your favourite luxury brand here) belt' is measurable and exciting. You may or may not have heard of 'vision boards'. They're commonly used as a tool to keep goals at the forefront of your mind. You find a range of visuals that match your goals, then stick them on a board on your wall, so you regularly see them. For example, my 2020 vision board was filled with images such as my completed book, a picture of a trophy with "10lbs lost" on it, a red vintage Mustang (my dream car), a bank transfer into my personal account featuring a £1 followed by a long series of zeros, and pictures of my family and me on fun holiday vacations.

Create your vision board and dream big and exciting. Add affirmations to your daily gratitude sessions, and make sure the things on your vision board are included. Throw off your limiting beliefs regarding whether or not you can achieve the items on your vision board and assume that you can succeed. Set many small goals, so you're ticking off achievements each day. Stay positive and use self-talk that's based in the future. In other words, don't say things like "I hope that I might succeed". Say, "I'm so thankful and grateful that success comes to me". It's vital you shake off any negative energy that you're carrying. Remember: all your thoughts trigger electrical and chemical responses in your brain that your chimp and subconscious mind respond to. Stay positive.

Start noticing as more and more things fall into place. This isn't a coincidence; it's your brain bringing external information to your conscious attention because it knows that information is relevant to your goals. The collection of neurons known as the reticular activating system play a fundamental role in this by deciding what to do with input from our senses through the brainstem. Tell your brain what your goals are, so it knows what information is relevant to achieving them.

The Law of Attraction that you may have heard of is based on these principles. If you set a clear purpose, align tangible, goal-based steps with that purpose, make sure your brain knows about them, and positively believe you can achieve them, the world can become a very exciting place. An Olympic athlete doesn't win a gold medal by telling their brain they probably can't succeed in this unlikely and difficult challenge. They win it by setting a clear purpose, aligning their goals towards it, frequently reminding their brain of the purpose and the goals, and repeatedly reminding their brain that they can and will achieve them. The great news is that these steps work for all of us, not just Olympic athletes.

9. I fixed my nutritional habits

I won't dive into detail here because I've covered this in chapter three, but I do urge you to remember that your gut is connected to your brain. There is a known network of nerve fibres connecting our intestinal cells with our nervous system. If you want to boost your brain function, your ability to make great decisions, and your ability to control your emotions and moods, then you must look after your microbiome. Feed yourself with lots of plant-based foods, get plenty of water, and practice intermittent fasting regularly to break your overeating habits. How you perceive your world, and your life, is undoubtedly influenced by the things you eat and drink. So, think very carefully about what you put into your system.

10. I used music

As always, I turned to music and sound extensively as one of my favoured, effective and versatile hacks. I used sound and music to fix my environment, as I explained previously. There are many ways to alter your environment and create an optimal environment. Light a candle to change the scent of a space, turn on a heater or fan to create a more comfortable temperature, sit in a more comfortable chair, adjust the lighting, and switch on some music. You can actually feed it directly into your ears to reduce the invasion of other sound information that might be picked up by your brain. The sound of other people or rain, for example. Once I've put my headphones on and started the music, the external world disappears. I've been taught how to quickly enter that flow state. If I'm working on something and listening to a soundscape, nothing is present except the laptop. I can get deeply immersed very quickly and get lots of work done in a short time. However, you need to find the type of soundscape or music playlist that works for you. Once you've found it, stick with it. I can't listen to any music that has words in it or things that are musically busy. I need floaty soundscapes that are almost empty but enough to keep my brain occupied so it doesn't distract me with other sounds in my environment. I created a soundscape I called a Focus Runway for this purpose. I've also been beta testing a machine-driven generative music platform. It's been designed for mental health therapy use, but I also believe it could have powerful uses to help people stay focused and keep on top of their workload, thereby managing work-related stress and poor mental health.

I've stayed away from playlists that are listed as "Focus playlists" on the usual streaming music platforms. After a lot of testing, I found that most of these playlists are not designed to help the brain focus and maintain attention. They are just playlists uploaded by people who have tagged them with the word 'focus' in the description, so they come up in searches. These playlists are better described as relaxation playlists than focused playlists. I found in most cases, they featured too much musical complexity and were distracting, even at low volume. I also used simplistic, relaxing soundscapes and playlists extensively during meditation and self-hypnosis sessions as they helped create the atmosphere I needed to achieve these mind states.

But it's not just about relaxation and slowing the brain down. I also regularly use music to induce an opposite effect when I need to achieve a fast spike of energy, enthusiasm and motivation. An up-tempo song that I can sing along with and dance to creates a simple and instant boost. I noticed that even when I'm doing this on my own, I tend to smile. While watching a Martin Scorsese documentary on Netflix recently, I heard his interviewee mention that a New York opera house now has cameras that pan across the audience during performances. The footage shows clearly how the audience naturally responds to music by smiling. I found the streaming music services very useful when I was looking for a song to give me a quick boost. The history of music is at my fingertips and can be called upon in an instant. It's amazing. In the afternoons, when I was trying to take more frequent breaks, I listened to vinyl. Streaming music goes on and on, so you can easily be sitting or standing still for hours. Whereas, when I put on a record, I have to break every 20-30 minutes to turn it over. It's a useful hack. Vinyl also makes me feel good because it triggers lots of positive memories from my youth. I feel as if I can achieve anything when I'm playing my vinyl collection.

Due to its position as an external sensory input, sound can play a massive part in how we experience life in positive and negative ways. In addition to the uses I've described above, there's a mountain of fascinating research happening around the world examining the use of music – and I'm deeply immersed in it. However, for the purposes of my experiment, I wanted to use music in a way that would be affordable for all and easy to access. So, I didn't use bio-tuning to find my optimal frequency or buy a vibroacoustic chair. However, I plan to delve much deeper into that area in my next book, the final edition of my health trilogy.

DIVE DEEPER

Here are some of my favourite books related to the concepts I explored in this chapter.

How Emotions Are Made by Lisa Feldman Barrett
The Secret Life of the Brain

Behave by Robert Sapolsky
The Biology of Humans at our Worst and Best

The Chimp Paradox by Professor Steve Peters

The Source by Dr Tara Swart
Open Your Mind. Change Your Life

The Brain by David Eagleman
The Story of You

Incognito by David Eagleman
The Secret Lives of the Brain

The Silva Mind Control Method by Jose Silva

Rest: Why You Get More Done When You Work Less by Alex Soojung-Kim Pang

Chapter 6

Moving

One in four adults, and four out of five adolescents, are not physically active enough. Globally this is estimated to cost US$54 billion in direct health care and US$14 billion in lost productivity
(World Health Organisation, 2020)

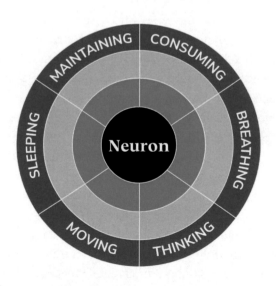

Note that the quote on the previous page says we're not "physically active enough", not that "we don't exercise enough". There's a difference. We do need to be physically active; we don't need to exercise. In my opinion, the word "exercise" has contributed to the poor state of health we see across the world today. As the exercise industry grew, we were led to believe that we need to be leaping around in gyms or exercise classes. In reality, as long as you're eating healthily and not overconsuming, you just need to get up and walk around more often to help your heart and lungs maintain their healthy working function. Even before the pandemic struck, confining us to lockdowns, most of us simply weren't moving enough. Some headlines offered a glimmer of hope in 2020, such as the surge in bicycle sales. However, on looking more closely, it was evident that those bicycle sales were driven by people buying electric bikes. Yes, the type of bikes that we can just sit on and let the motor do the work. Decades of health promotions telling us all to move more have not worked. I've spent a lifetime trying to encourage people to be more active and also trying to figure out why they don't do it. No one wants to be unhealthy, and everyone knows they need to be more active to avoid that poor health destiny. So why on earth is it so difficult to achieve? The answer, as usual, lies largely in our brain.

As discussed earlier, our ancient hunter-gatherer ancestors moved because it was part of survival. They moved to gather food, to build and maintain shelter, to look after children and various other tasks. They didn't need exercise routines or gyms. Physical movement happened naturally because of the tasks and actions they completed each day to maintain life. Modern society has removed that type of routine from us. We've spent over 100 years inventing labour-saving techniques and innovations that enable us to move as little as possible. So now we have to actually choose to move in order to prevent the inevitable decline of our brains and bodies. However, as we can clearly see from the identified health trends, exercise classes, gyms, and treadmills aren't the answer. Our brain doesn't view them as necessary for survival. So, we have to force ourselves to maintain these unnatural acts.

I've found myself moving less and less in recent years. Despite being a member of a gym, I rarely entered the building. It was simply too time intensive, requiring me to travel to and from the destination, navigate traffic, park, sign in, change into exercise clothing and find a locker, head to the gym to see what equipment was free, warm-up, do 20-30 minutes of actual exercise, shower etc. The entire palaver cost almost two hours of my day. That's simply too much lost time for most people, and frankly, it's a waste of time. You don't need to go to a gym or an exercise class to maintain good health.

For my experiment, I vowed to remind myself of the key science and to employ hacks to maintain the maximum effects of physical activity with the minimum effort and time cost.

What do we actually need to do physically?

I don't like wasting time, so I wanted to figure out what the 'minimum viable product' was when it came to physical activity and maintain basic wellness. I know that's not what the fitness and exercise industry tries to convince us to do. Science shows our cells start to degrade in our early adult years. Our environment and behaviour through our lifetime can either speed up that process of decline or slow it down. Most of us are speeding it up due to our poor habits and choices. We're also surrounded by an environment that pushes us towards inactivity. If you have a desk job, the situation is even worse, and remote working fuelled by Covid-19 has further amplified the danger of extended periods of inactivity. This has other hidden dangers. For example, physical movement helps stimulate the transit of food through the digestive system. An overeating habit, plus an addiction to unhealthy food, plus inactivity, led to a boom in laxative sales over the years.

   The further I dug into the science, the more I realised how important our muscle tissue is. It's massively overlooked in general public health campaigns. They tend to focus on leaping around in exercise gear. This type of activity is also promoted as a route to weight loss, but in reality, physical activity doesn't impact energy burn significantly enough to be a major fat loss driver. If you have fat to lose, you need to focus on fixing your overeating and poor nutrition habits. Head back to the information I presented in chapter 3 to remind yourself how to get rid of your excess fat stores. Then come back here to learn how to increase the efficiency of your metabolic pathways through your muscle tissue, to ensure that fat accumulation never happens again.

It was only after speaking with medical physician and strength guru, Dr Doug McGuff, that the penny really dropped in my mind about the importance of muscles. But before I get to that, let's do a quick summary of the science. I majored in exercise physiology in both my undergraduate and master's degrees, so I have a pretty detailed understanding of the anatomical and physiological underpinnings of activity. I also studied biomechanics, so I have a solid understanding of the efficiency of movement. However, it's only when you add in the additional brain and nervous system elements that the full picture emerges – and, as usual, it stems from our ancient survival responses.

Muscles need to be engaged very quickly and at a high intensity if we need to rapidly evacuate from a threat environment. When the brain detects what it thinks is a dangerous situation, it triggers action potentials in the neurons in our motor cortex (part of the frontal lobe of the brain). The action potentials travel along the axon of the neurons to our muscles. When they reach the muscle cells, acetylcholine is released from the end of the axon, triggering the activation of the muscle fibres. The muscles are attached to our bones, so when the muscle fibres leap into action, we're able to very quickly move away from trouble and survive another day. This whole process is fuelled by food nutrients and oxygen.

The key thing to remember is that our muscles are far more important than most of us realise. They dictate many other processes that determine our wellness, including our immunity and our fat stores due to core metabolic processes and the muscle-derived production of proteins and hormones that modulate them. Putting your muscles under a load (a stressor) not only helps to reduce the age-related decline of muscle tissue, it also triggers growth hormone activity that extends beyond our muscles.

Of course, these days, we don't often find ourselves in a situation where we need to engage that fight or flight movement to escape a predator. So, we need to fake it. This is where biohacking principles can step in and transform your health. For my experiment, I realised I needed to mimic our ancestors by doing a few high-intensity sprints each week (check with your doctor before doing high-intensity work if you think you may have an underlying cause for concern), lots of walking and some lifting that overloaded my muscles. Here's how I employed various hacks in my experiment:

My Top Moving Hacks

1. I focused on efficiency (less is more)

Most of the exercise recommendations we're given by fitness brands and health organisations are a waste of time. They're highly inefficient activities based on outdated ideas maintained because the fitness industry makes money from them. For example, do you need to go to a gym to maintain physical health? No. Do you need an exercise class? No. Does an exercise class need to last 45 mins to an hour? No. Do you need exercise equipment? No. I could make this list much longer, but I'm sure you get the picture. The simple fact is that decades ago, we built a fitness industry (I include myself in this 'we'), based on some basic ideas and science that we now know were quite flawed. Sessions were structured on basic scheduling ideas ("We'll make these sessions 30 mins or 60 mins because that seems like a round number and fit well into this booking system/software"). They failed to produce a healthy nation for a reason. Our inner chimp does not see these long, repetitive sessions as necessary for survival. However, they became so ingrained in society that they are still being promoted today as health solutions. The problem is they're highly ineffective and time-consuming, and they do not align with our evolutionary brain and body circuits. So, for most people, these types of fitness regimes are impossible to stick to. This, of course, is why the fitness industry business model is so financially successful. We're told to join a gym to improve our health, so we dutifully do, but we hardly ever make it there and take ages to finally cancel our direct debit payments. It happens every January. Don't get me wrong, if you enjoy going to a gym or exercise class, you're getting a health benefit from it. If you want to achieve significant fitness scores (over and above what you need to simply maintain basic wellness), then the gym is also an asset that can help you achieve that goal because the machines help you push past the limit of what you can achieve with your own bodyweight. However, if like me, you just want to avoid poor health and maintain basic wellness until the age of 100, you don't need any of those things. You need efficiency. You need habits that produce sufficient results with the minimum time and effort. Efficiency became my focus, and the facts became clear – less is more. The key is simply to trigger our in-built adaptive response. In other words, engage our brain, nervous system and basic biology. So I started doing less.

2. I made 'adaptive response' my supertool

In the same way that our brain cells alter continuously in response to environmental stimuli, our muscles also alter after they're put in a stressful situation. The unusual sudden stimulus tells the brain that some sort of external stressor put us under pressure, and it may have been something that was a threat to our survival — for example, having to lift a fallen tree off our leg or run away from a predator. This signals a range of changes that are designed to ensure that those muscle fibres are stronger and more capable of rapidly fuelling movement if that situation happens again. If the muscle fibres never experience this type of stress (i.e. because we're inactive and live in a safe environment), our cells gradually deteriorate, and we lose muscle tissue.

This adaptive response is very important because it isn't just linked to our ability to run faster or lift tree trunks. The changes that occur in our muscle cells also send signalling molecules to other tissues in our body that affect our metabolism and immune system. If we're inactive, it's not just our muscles that suffer; it's our entire body. This is why inactivity is linked to so many chronic diseases and inflammation. It's vital to build and maintain muscle tissue. To achieve this state, I realised I needed to regularly do movements that required a lot of fuel in a short space of time. I needed to do things that took me to exhaustion. When you reach that point, you can be confident your glucose-hungry muscles have depleted the available glycogen stores. Your brain knows something has to be done in response to this sudden serious situation.

3. I used my autonomic nervous system

To trigger a fight or flight sympathetic response, I needed movements that resembled a sudden threat. I found a hill near my home with long steep steps and sprinted full pelt to the top. This definitely brought me to exhaustion. Near the top, I can hardly keep going. My legs turn to jelly. I have to start using my hands on my knees to keep pushing my legs into motion. I have to stand still when I reach the summit because my legs feel so weak I worry they might buckle. At this point, I can feel reasonably confident that my muscles have hoovered through my glycogen stores. It's taken approximately 30-40 seconds to get to the top. As I slowly walk back down the steps, my body will be quickly replacing those stores in case I need to run from that imaginary tiger again. It's a remarkable feature of our body that just a few minutes after we simply cannot move another step, we can begin to do so again. So, up I go again at full throttle. The second time it's harder.

In the past, based on outdated models of what a "training session" should be, I'd probably have continued doing lots of these sprints. This is what instructors are still making people do (I regularly do' mystery shopper' visits to gyms and fitness classes to see what is being sold and recommended to people). However, the reality is that just doing one or two of these 30-40 second sprints a couple of times a week is sufficient to maintain wellness. It puts your heart, lungs and muscles into a survival scenario and triggers an adaptive response to ensure your muscle tissue is maintained. The problem is that a fitness class that only lasts a few minutes would be tough to price. So, they don't exist. If a traditional 30- to 60-minute exercise class today costs £5, how much would you pay for one that lasted less than 5 minutes – the time it takes me to do two sprints up my steps?

Partway through my experiment, I discovered a new exercise bicycle called Car. OL. It stands for cardiovascular optimisation logic. The bike uses artificial intelligence technology to learn how your body responds to resistance. It then calibrates your ride, increasing the resistance during a 20-second sprint so that by the 20th second, you can hardly move your legs. It takes you to exhaustion through rapid glycogen depletion. After a few minutes of gentle cycling and low slow 4:6 ratio breathing (close to my resonance frequency – see chapter 4), you sprint again for 20 seconds. The concept is aimed at triggering the body's natural adaptive response, improving your insulin response (getting glucose into the muscle cells), improving the efficiency of your metabolism (delivering oxygen and glucose and removing waste products) and building healthy muscle tissue. The breathing exercises and the narrated soundtrack are designed to actively engage your autonomic nervous system, switching it between sudden sympathetic fight or flight mode during the sprints, then back into a relaxed parasympathetic mode with controlled breathing during the slower recovery periods between the two sprints. According to the peer-reviewed studies, the two 20-second sprints can deliver the equivalent benefit of a 45-minute run. Doing this twice a week is all that's needed. What I particularly liked about this bike is that the intense sprints happen so fast your body doesn't have time to get hot. So, you don't sweat, and you don't need to change into exercise gear or have a shower. It's a highly efficient method. The start of the sprint is simple, and then the resistance kicks in. I couldn't replicate this when running up the steps. The size of the steps and incline are relatively equal throughout. So, it takes longer to reach the point of exhaustion, and I end up with a hot, sweaty face because my body temperature has risen. The Car. OL bike isn't accessible to everyone because it's pretty expensive (approximately £3,000 at the time of writing).

4. I used slow-motion for strength

So now you know that rapid glycogen depletion is a vital goal. This is what kicks our evolutionary adaptive survival responses into action. Maintaining strength is key. As well as pretending to sprint away from a tiger, you can also achieve glycogen depletion through slow-motion movements that take muscle groups to the point of exhaustion. It's valuable to add these into your week because it means you can focus on all main muscle groups. Whereas your sprints are mostly just stressing your leg muscles.

I added strength work to make sure my upper body was included. I used push-ups, but I also bought a barbell so I could add some squats and deadlifts for my legs. However, I mostly used the barbell and push-ups because my step sprints (and then the Car. OL bike were enough for my legs).

For push-ups (or barbell chest presses), I simply did slow-motion movement up and down until my muscles were not able to continue. Approaching the point of exhaustion, you'll be shaking like a jelly and probably making some Neanderthal grunting noises. Well done, you've achieved glycogen depletion in your chest and arm muscles. During your push-ups, your other muscles are also working hard to maintain your core position. For extra efficiency in overloading your muscles, spend more time on the downward phase of the movement to stress your muscle fibres when they are lengthening (eccentric) than the upward phase (concentric). The slow-motion rate is important because it means the effect of momentum never reaches a point where the load on the muscle fibres is slightly eased. If you're moving fast, momentum assists as you overcome gravity. It's like throwing a ball in the air. When it leaves your hand, it keeps going. The same happens with your body. If you quickly push it away from the floor, your muscles are not continually under maximum load. If you push your bodyweight away from the floor more slowly, you'll reach the point of exhaustion sooner. Don't stop between the up and down phase.

Ensure the movement is slow, continuous and fluid until you absolutely can no longer do it.

There is a lot more detail regarding the precise tempo of the eccentric and concentric phases, but for the purposes of my experiment, I was simply aiming to grow and maintain a healthy level of muscle tissue and metabolic efficiency. I wasn't aiming to build a significantly greater mass of muscle through a major hypertrophic response, or do body sculpting. Simple slow-motion exercises for a few minutes twice a week was enough for my goals. I noticed the difference in general strength within a few weeks.

It's important to remember that muscle groups work in pairs. So just doing push-ups is not going to be beneficial in the long-term. It will create an imbalance, making one set of muscles stronger than their counterpart. In the case of push-ups, they work the chest and triceps (back of arm) muscles but not the opposite muscles in your back and biceps (front of arm). So, to work in those regions, I bought a resistance band. I hooked it over a door and pulled down on the ends using slow-motion movement. This enabled me to raise and lower my hands with even resistance. If you're not doing leg work through sprints, you can add a slow-motion drop by squatting down onto a chair (don't let your bum touch it) to work the front muscles of your legs, and add a leg curl to work the back muscles of your legs (using the resistance band and squeezing your foot up towards your bum).

The key is to keep it slow and steady until you deplete the muscles fuel stores and reach exhaustion. This slow-motion pace also helps reduce the risk of injury.

Everyone should be doing basic strength work to maintain muscle tissue throughout life and prevent the decline of vital cells as we age. There is still a huge misconception, particularly among older women, that strength training isn't for them. Let's bust this myth right now. Your muscles play a major role in your ability to control bodyweight and also participate in the health of your immune system responses, your bone health and more.

5. I harnessed optic flow and the power of walking

I'm a big fan of walking. Our ancient ancestors walked a lot to stay alive, gather food and find shelter. We're designed to efficiently do two main types of physical activity necessary for survival: sprint away from life-threatening situations and walk for long periods when safe. The glycogen-depleting movements I've described mimic the survival sprints. In addition, I needed to walk. Being a dog owner, this wasn't difficult for me.

Walking involves every muscle in the body and our metabolic pathways and cardiorespiratory systems. However, I discovered additional benefits that I wasn't aware of. For instance, an effect called 'optic flow' happens as our eyes take in the natural environment in our periphery. This effect is part of the ancient parasympathetic response and elicits a relaxation response. This forward motion doesn't happen when you're walking on a treadmill in a gym with your eyes focused on a TV screen throwing blue light at you. In fact, your eyes are more likely to be in sympathetic stress mode in that scenario. So, walking outdoors is an effective wellness tool.

6. I identified causes of pain and made changes

Most of us put up with aches and pains, doing nothing about them until they reach a point where there's a crisis, and we're in such pain that we have to do something. Sometimes that delay is due to the cost of therapy or purely the inconvenience of having to book and attend appointments. I've been noticing a very sore right hip for about 10 months. It's been getting worse. It only happens when I wake up and then disappears throughout the day. I've been trying various stretches but couldn't seem to hit the precise spot with them. So, I eventually got a diagnosis. It turns out to be my piriformis. My hip rotators (a group of muscles that rotate your leg) are not balanced. Some are weaker than others, and that's put extra strain on my piriformis. Once the problem was identified, I could find the stretches and exercises that targeted the issue and rebalance the muscles. However, I wanted to know why this had happened, so I examined my daily activity to see what habits might be causing it. I realised that in the morning, I sit in my favourite chair while I do some deep focused writing and reading. I sit with my legs crossed in this position for fairly long periods. This results in my right leg being twisted, with the weight of the other one on top of it. As soon as I'd identified this, I made a point of stopping the leg-crossing habit.

I also ordered a stand-up desk and an anti-fatigue mat, so I spent less time sitting in the chair. Plus, I adjusted my coffee habit. In the morning, I used to pour my coffee into my largest mug (it's huge). I replaced it with a smaller one, forcing me to get out of my chair more often to refill it. I now make four or five trips to the kitchen instead of two. This has broken up the amount of time I'm sitting still in the morning. Changing my mug also helped me break the leg-crossing habit because I was getting up more. I also put the printer upstairs to increase the number of times I went up the steps. So far, so good, the sore hip problem appears to be fixed. Using your environment to initiate movement is an easy way to increase your activity. Don't organise it in a way that reduces your movement; organise it in a way that requires movement.

7. I fixed my nutrition and my sleep

I won't go into detail on this one as we covered it in other chapters. However, your nutrition is highly linked to your movement because it's your fuel. Sleep is also highly linked to your general energy level. All these elements are related. Improve your nutrition, and your energy will increase, resulting in improvements in your metabolism. Your sleep will improve, and that will, in turn, further increase your physical movement because you'll naturally have more energy and won't feel as tired.

8. I used nasal breathing to boost the relaxation effect

The breathing techniques I outlined in chapter 4 were also embedded into my physical activity routine. I consciously stopped my habitual mouth breathing during my walks and maintained an easy-paced low and slow breathing using my nose for inhalation (and exhalation if possible). I also used it in between sprints to engage the relaxation response.

9. I increased my interest using tech and measurements

As with my other biohacks, I embraced technology. There is a vast array of affordable devices that can track your movement and give readings about your activity level and heart rate. Using these basic measurements helps make your walks more enjoyable. You see what happens to your heart rate when you add hills or increase your pace. You can get a little buzz of excitement when your smartwatch or tracker celebrates hitting your step goal. It's an easy way to stay motivated.

10. I used music

There are many positive ways music can help increase your physical activity and boost your motivation to move. I began researching this field in the 1990s. Music is a superb biohack and helps influence your brain activity and chemical secretion. However, if you're running, I realised that my typical use of music could complicate the use of breathwork. Impact stress is believed to be at its greatest when your footstrike happens at the moment you begin an exhalation. At this moment of exhaling, your diaphragm and associated core muscles are relaxing; this decreases the internal stability just at the moment of impact. If you're running using an even breathing rhythm timed with the music, this means that you're always landing on the same foot during an exhalation, for example, breathing in for two steps and out for two steps. This can lead to repetitive injury if you're engaging in this for prolonged periods. The ideal breathing rhythm is one that results in alternating footstrikes during exhales. For example, three steps for an inhale and two steps during exhale. This enables you to alternate the side you footstrike during exhale. Breathing at this rhythm would be confusing to embed if you're using a standard music playlist that features an even tempo (most popular music playlists). So, either practice it without music or use soundscapes that do not feature a regular and repeating rhythm.

Music and sound also played a major role in the Car. OL bike sessions: helping create a sense of threat during the sprint sessions and safety during the recovery periods. I also used vinyl a lot because it got me out of my chair regularly to turn the record over. Our body naturally moves to music, so it's a very effective biohack.

DIVE DEEPER

Here are a few recommended reads if you're interested in delving deeper into this topic.

Body by Science by Doug McGuff, MD.

Exercised by Daniel Lieberman
The Science of Physical Activity, Rest and Health

Chapter 7

Sleeping

One of the most important parts of your day is actually at night. Sleep is an essential pillar of health. It's the time when your brain carries out necessary housekeeping and maintenance

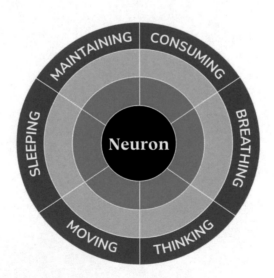

As my experiment progressed, it became abundantly clear that true wellness can only really be achieved if you master every aspect. For example, the food and drink you consume impacts pretty much everything. So does your movement. Your sleep quality does too. See below for an example of what happens to my heart rate variability scores when I have just one night of poor quality sleep. You'll remember that in the chapter on breathing, I showed you how I'd improved the general health of my autonomic nervous system to the point of consistently achieving high heart rate variability (HRV) scores. However, in the chart below, you can see that poor sleep produces a drop in my morning HRV score and shows a slight dominance of the sympathetic (stress response) nervous system. I woke up feeling tired on this day. I'd had naughty food and a couple of large glasses of wine the night before.

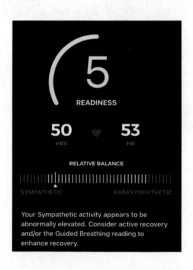

After a few days of getting back into my good habits, my sleep patterns re-settled, and my baseline morning HRV scores returned to my normal higher, healthier level, as you can see below.

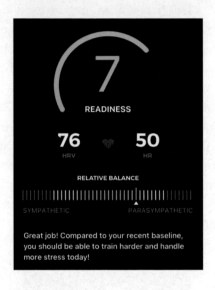

Consistently good quality sleep eludes many people. It's something we all want but sometimes is hard to achieve due to modern lifestyles. We're doing the wrong things. When I started my experiment, I knew that I frequently went to bed too late, ate my food too late, and used screens too late – all things you shouldn't do. I also knew that poor sleep throughout adult life probably damages neurons. Having a bit of a lie-in on a Sunday doesn't fix the problem. In fact, it makes it worse, as you'll see in later pages. Poor sleep through adulthood is now considered a contributing factor in the accelerated decline of brain tissue. The damage begins decades before symptoms become apparent. So, pay careful attention to this chapter to help reduce your risk of dementia in later life.

Let's start by looking at our hunter-gatherer relatives again. A recent study mentioned that the few remaining hunter-gatherer tribes don't actually have a word that describes *insomnia* in their language because they don't experience it. That is very illuminating. Our 'Western' cultural modern life messes up our sleep. Hunter-gatherer communities reportedly sleep on average 6.5 hours per night. That's slightly less than our current recommended range of 7-9 hours per night. However, they sleep well. 6.5 hours per night is the average that I usually manage to get. It's not just about the amount of sleep you clock up, though; quality is also vital. There are distinct phases our brain needs to cycle through during sleep to maintain our cells' health and function. We'll talk more about these cycles later.

How does sleep work?

Human sleep patterns are regulated by the light received by our eyes. If you want to fix your sleep, you need to make a note of that fact. Light entering the eye is detected by light-sensitive cells at the back of the eye in an area called the retina. This triggers electrochemical action potentials that travel from the retina, along the nerve fibres, to neurons in the brain. The retina can also detect where that light is coming from. In the case of daylight, it comes from above us (the sun). Our evolutionary sleep habits enabled us to do tasks necessary for survival when it was light enough to see, then rest during the night when it wasn't light enough. You'd imagine that through evolution, sleep would have been phased out because logic would suggest that sleeping at any time makes us vulnerable to predators. But even predators have to sleep. It's a vital part of our existence. Our ancestors who slept well survived because their sleep habits enabled them to function well when awake. Of course, they also found ways to stay safe while they were asleep. They formed communities and took it in turns to keep watch over each other's safety overnight; they built shelters to protect themselves from predators and used fire to keep unwanted visitors at bay.

So, we know that sleep is vital to survival. We spend a third of our day asleep – that's a third of your life. If you live to the age of 90, you'll have been asleep for 30 years of it. We also know that light is the key to healthy sleep patterns. The light-activated signals received by the retina inform a tiny region of neurons in the hypothalamus called the suprachiasmatic nuclei (a great name for a band, I think). These neurons act as the main control switch for our rhythms of sleep. This synchronising activity is known as our *circadian rhythm* or *circadian clock*. It's a master timer that sends messages to other parts of the brain and body. Inside the cells of the suprachiasmatic nuclei, a cycle of protein expression and degradation occurs. This cycle takes approximately 24 hours.

The suprachiasmatic nuclei cells are connected to a small structure called the pineal gland. During the daytime, the suprachiasmatic nuclei act as a brake on the pineal gland, inhibiting its activity. When active, the pineal gland makes a hormone called melatonin and releases it into the bloodstream. This chemical is involved in many responses, including adjustments in our body temperature and blood pressure. Melatonin is sometimes called the 'hormone of darkness' because that's when it gets to work. When the light fades and darkness falls, the pineal gland releases melatonin into our bloodstream. The rising levels cause drowsiness during the evening. The levels increase during the night as we sleep. The 24-hour cycle begins again when the retinal cells in our eyes once again sense light the next morning. This internal biological timer is so sensitive it can detect changes in the seasons due to the length of the daylight hours shortening and lengthening. Travelling large distances disrupts this sensitive clock and results in disturbed sleep, which we're all familiar with as 'jet lag'. Taking a melatonin supplement and getting exposure to light can help reset this temporary disruption.

What are sleep cycles?

Sleep isn't 'lost time'. The brain is busy while we sleep. We generally cycle through phases featuring two types of sleep: rapid eye movement (REM) and non-REM

(NREM). NREM has three stages. Stage 1 NREM is a short period of light sleep as you drift from wakefulness into sleep. Your breathing, heart rate, eye movement and muscle activity slows as you relax. Electrical activity in your brain starts to slow down. Stage 2 NREM is another period of light sleep and is repeated several times during the night as you cycle between deeper sleep and REM sleep. During this stage 2 sleep, you relax further. Stage 3 NREM is the deepest stage of sleep. It occurs during the first half of your night's sleep. Brainwaves are at their slowest (called delta waves), as is your heart rate and breathing. It's difficult to wake someone when they are in this deep sleep stage.

In contrast to the NREM sleep stages, REM sleep features rapid eye movement behind your closed eyelids (hence the name) and increased brain activity. Dreaming occurs during REM sleep. The brain deactivates the muscles in your legs and arms during this stage so that you don't act out your dreams. Blood pressure, breathing and heart rate are also higher during REM sleep than in other phases. Most of your REM sleep happens in the second half of your night.

The deeper sleep stages feature important maintenance processes, including the calibration of cardiovascular physiology and removing excess toxins that build up over time. These toxins are linked with Alzheimer's disease if they continue to accumulate over the years. Deep sleep gets a lot of attention due to its cleansing properties. But REM sleep is now known to be important too. It is believed to be the stage where we process emotional memories. There is a lot of heart rate variability during REM sleep as our cardiovascular system cycles between periods of activation and rest. When REM sleep is consistently impaired, a person can experience stress and anxiety. So, REM sleep seems to provide an important emotionally therapeutic role. It helps us process memories, learn to deal with stressful events, and assists with the regulation of mood-associated brain chemicals during waking hours.

Be aware that your brain never really manages to properly catch up on lost sleep, known as sleep debt. It will try, but as well as the work that wasn't completed during the previous night of lost sleep, it also has the additional new tasks to complete. In studies, when people are deprived of sleep for 24 hours or more, their brain tries hard to recoup the lost hours. Typically, on the first night of sleep after a period of deprivation, they sleep for much longer than usual. During the first night, they will experience higher amounts of NREM deep sleep. On subsequent nights they will experience increased levels of REM sleep. So, the brain seems to prioritise NREM sleep in this situation. One night of disrupted or lost sleep can negatively impact your rhythm for several days.

As outlined in previous chapters, the steps I took automatically helped improve my sleep during my experiment. My greatly improved eating and drinking habits, combined with daily moderate physical activity, helped my brain maintain a steady circadian rhythm. On the following pages, you'll see the hacks and changes to my routine I added to help embed good habits to support sleep. My sleep architecture improved (the shape and consistency of the cycles), but I'd still like to increase my average sleep time from 6.5 hours per night to above 7 hours. It's a work in progress. I choose to get up early because that's when my brain can do its most focused work. I'm highly productive in the morning between 6am and midday. However, that means I'd need to head to bed at 9.30pm or 10pm to get sufficient sleep. Sometimes I achieve that, but not every night.

My Top Sleeping Hacks

1. I paid a lot of attention to light

Once I realised how vital natural daylight is to the internal master clock, I specifically embedded new habits to maintain and strengthen that synchronisation effect. My old wake-up routine involved getting out of bed and letting my dog out into the garden. I used to open the door and let him out, but I would stay inside in the warm. This meant that sometimes I was indoors for several more hours before I left the house. I decided to embed a new habit of physically going outside into the garden with my dog instead of just opening the door for him. This meant I got light in my eyes before 6.30am instead of the usual time I left the house, hours later. You don't need to look at the sun (that's dangerously damaging to your eyes), just being outside in the natural light is sufficient to tell your brain morning has arrived. I also made sure I was out again at sunset so that my suprachiasmatic nuclei got an extra boost of natural light dusk information so it would maintain a strong calibration. In theory, approximately 16 hours after your eyes sense light in the morning, your chemical clock should ensure that an 8-hour sleep period starts. It's important to note that indoor light is nowhere close to being as powerful as sunlight. So, throw open a window and stick your head out for some morning light if you don't have a garden.

Once I'd established the routine to maximise the effect of natural light, I also needed to ensure there was nothing unnatural in my routine that messed it up. During the day, the spectrum of natural daylight changes. By the time sunset is approaching, the amount of blue light in natural light is greatly reduced. However, we invented light bulbs and technology featuring screens, and they all emit lots of blue light. Our retina would only usually be sensing this much blue light during the daytime. So, it's mightily confusing to your brain if you're shining blue light in there at night. To solve this problem, I used dimmer switches to ensure my indoor lighting during the evening was not bright. I also bought some dimmer table lamps, so the lighting was below my eye level even when I was sitting on the sofa. Remember, your retina can sense which direction the light is coming from, so if you have bright ceiling lights switched on above you at night, your brain interprets that as sunlight. It's better to switch them off and use low-height table lamps or buy a dimmer switch. Candles are also good. To counteract the blue light from my smartphone and computer screens in the evening, I bought a pair of glasses designed to block blue light. I also set a timer on my phone that prevented me from using apps after 9pm. In the end, I decided the timer was more effective than using blue-blocking glasses at preventing my late-night screen habit.

2. I created an optimal sleep environment

We already know from previous chapters that the brain takes in external information from our surroundings, even when we're not consciously aware of it. So it makes good sense to think hard about your bedroom. After doing a basic evaluation, I realised I could make several changes. I removed all piles of books and paperwork. I decluttered all surfaces. I adjusted the radiator so the room wouldn't get too hot (a cooler environment is more conducive to sleep because it reflects how the temperature drops at night in a natural outdoor setting). I used a scented candle to create a specific smell that I used as a cue for bedtime. I also put some drops of aromatherapy oil on my skin. I set up a radio with a timer feature. I also bought small dimmer lights with a timer feature, so once I was in bed, they gradually switched themselves off one by one until I was in complete darkness. I made sure my pillows felt comfortable. I created a room that is lovely to visit. It's an experiential sleep zone rather than just a room in the house where I sleep. It's a pleasure to head to. The habit of making my bed in the morning to boost dopamine and serotonin also yields extra benefits at night because the bed is tidy and inviting when I arrive for sleep.

If you need additional help, other suggestions include blackout curtains, little stickers to put over any visible LED light dots on devices, acoustic dampeners on your walls to help create a sleep pod vibe, acoustic curtains, blindfolds, and earplugs.

3. *I stopped using my phone as an alarm*

Using the alarm feature on your smartphone is a really detrimental habit if you're trying to improve your sleep. It means you often have your phone in your hand when you climb into bed. Not only is this emitting blue light, but it's also increasing the likelihood that the highly addictive social media apps will lure you in. Switch it off. Leave it downstairs if you can. Don't use it as an alarm clock. I set my radio to be the alarm instead. Although, once I got into my routine, I found that my sleep timing was so consistent that I was waking up without the need for an alarm clock. Lockdown helped test this out because it gave me the confidence not to set an alarm. It didn't matter if I accidentally slept late because I didn't have to be anywhere.

4. *I added breathwork to my bedtime routine*

Resting heart rate and breathing rate decreases when you drift into the sleep stages. So, I tried increasing the likelihood of this by starting the process myself before falling asleep. I used the breathing techniques described in chapter 4 to take my regular breathing down low and slow towards my resonance frequency. I started this routine while brushing my teeth.

5. I bought a weighted blanket

The effects of deep pressure are known to be capable of stimulating calming responses. A comforting hug from a parent or being swaddled in clothing when young elicits a relaxation and safety response. In recent years, weighted blankets have become increasingly popular as a tool to improve sleep. The belief is that the weight of the heavy blanket simulates these effects and increases the parasympathetic arousal of the autonomic nervous system, reducing sympathetic activation (inhibiting a stress response and boosting a relaxation response). There have been positive results seen in sleep improvement and anxiety reduction. I bought one to try for myself. The pandemic brought care requirements that resulted in our family being separated. So, I found myself suddenly sleeping alone. I absolutely loved the weighted blanket from the outset. It perhaps helps that it arrived during winter, so it adds an extra level of cosiness as well as the weight. I've been sleeping exceptionally well since I started using it. Although, in retrospect, it is probably too heavy for me. When initially doing my research, I was on a forum where many people were discussing their blankets, many of whom were mentioning a 20lb blanket. So, in my haste to make a purchase, that's what I ordered. I later discovered that you should actually buy one that's

10% of your body weight. I should really have bought a 13lb blanket.

6. I switched to decaf after 2pm

I'm a coffee fan. When used properly, it has health benefits, as we discussed in chapter 3. However, caffeine molecules bind (like a lock and key) to receptors on the outer membrane of the neurons that are designed to receive a brain chemical called adenosine. Like melatonin, as adenosine levels rise and increase their braking effect on neurons, it eventually results in sleepiness. It inhibits activity in neurons that are involved in arousal and wakefulness. However, caffeine molecules are structurally very similar to adenosine molecules, so they can fit and bind to the adenosine receptors on neurons' cell membrane. However, they don't produce the same effect on the neurons as adenosine. They just act as a block on the receptor. Consequently, adenosine cannot exert its inhibitory influence on those neurons. So, we continue to feel awake until those caffeine molecules are removed. This process can take hours. This effect makes caffeine known as an *adenosine antagonist*. It also enhances the activation of our sympathetic nervous system (fight/flight/freeze), giving us an energy boost. However, it also produces dopamine in our reward pathways and can become addictive if consumed too frequently in large doses. I found that as well as improving my sleep, a switch to decaf coffee in the afternoon reduced its addictive impact.

7. I removed evening access to phone apps

Dimming my light bulbs helped reduce the amount of blue light exposure at night. Also, I tried to restrict the use of my phone and laptop in the evenings. This is not a good habit to have. I find social media apps the worst culprits. They are specifically designed to trigger your addictive dopamine reward pathways. Hours can be lost scrolling mindlessly through pages of content. I moved my social media apps off the home screen of my phone and switched off notifications. The immediate silence was noticeable. This did mean that I lost contact with people, but it's a trade-off. Do I really need to be connected with this many people several times a day? Probably not. I also set a timer on my phone so that it no longer gave those apps access to Wi-Fi after 8pm. I could over-ride it if I wanted to, but it at least acted as a barrier to entry. My social media use greatly reduced during my experiment. I don't miss it at all.

8. I used self-hypnosis/meditation to enter a trance state

Getting into a sleep mindset when climbing into bed is a hugely valuable part of the journey to good sleep. As well as fixing my sleep environment to create an enjoyable external space, I also focussed on creating an internal environment that was conducive to sleep. It's not helpful to lie in bed stressing about things. If there's a lot on your mind, keep a note pad by your bed and write them down, so they are out of your mind.

I used guided meditation and self-hypnosis recordings every night when I began my experiment. Now I continue to use them occasionally, but I am so good at falling asleep I don't need them as much. If you're struggling to get to sleep due to a racing mind, I would highly recommend this approach. It's an easy way to slow down your brain activity and get to know your inner mind and subconscious brain. Remember, regular good sleep makes it much easier to stay in control and make good decisions during your waking hours. Good habits are harder to maintain when you're tired and weak. So, use guided meditation and self-hypnosis recordings to build a strong mindset, visualise clear goals, and achieve superb sleep quality. The more often you practice these techniques, the easier it becomes to enter this trance-like state where you're floating between consciousness and sleep.

9. I used tech to monitor my sleep quality

I find it greatly helps me maintain a new habit if I measure it. This daily act of recording makes the whole process more enjoyable. It also helps me to see how my actions during the day impact my physiology. Sleep is no exception. I used my FitBit to monitor my sleep activity, and you can see some of my typical sleep scores below. My sleep quality improved greatly during my experiment, but I'd still like to increase my average night's sleep to seven hours if I can. I also found it interesting to see that when I awoke from a very vivid dream, it was because I emerged out of a long period of REM sleep. My heart rate during sleep was much less frantic during the nights that I used guided meditation or self-hypnosis to get into trance mode before drifting off. Heart rate should resemble a hammock during sleep: gradually dropping and then increasing. Monitoring this information using trackers and apps can help you bring the science to life and see it in action.

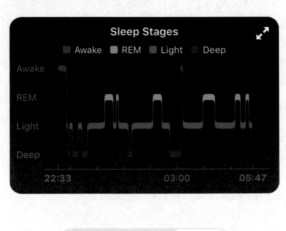

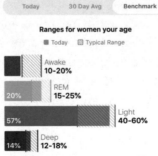

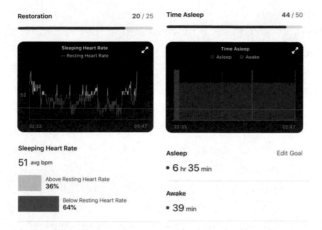

Restoration   20 / 25   **Time Asleep**   44 / 50

Sleeping Heart Rate

51 avg bpm

Above Resting Heart Rate
36%

Below Resting Heart Rate
64%

Asleep   Edit Goal

• 6 hr 35 min

Awake

• 39 min

10. I used music

Music before sleep works best if it helps reassure your brain that you are safe. Low volume, slow tempo, music that makes you feel good in some way is a great addition to your evening. It helps get you on the early stages of the sleep runway, increasing the likelihood of good quality sleep. It doesn't really matter what music it is as long as it makes you feel relaxed and doesn't trigger your sympathetic nervous system. Many people watch high-action, loud movies and TV before heading straight to bed. They then wonder why they can't sleep. Your goal is to reduce the activation of your sympathetic nervous system, not trigger an adrenaline response. So, switch off the TV and put on some music that you find calming.

Keep playing it through your night-time routine as you get ready for bed.

Music *for* sleep gets a lot of attention, but in reality, there is no specific sound that's going to be guaranteed to send you to sleep. It's a highly individual experience, and you need to find the type of playlist or soundscape that works best for you. Sleep also depends on many other factors such as the type of evening you've had, the level of activity in your brain and the state of your autonomic nervous system.

However, there are general principles that help narrow the search. Sounds that are relaxing are more likely to give your brain that reassuring message. Calming sounds of nature can also work. Your brain can't stop itself from translating language when it hears words. So, if you're using music with human vocals, that's probably not helping. The exception to this rule is the vocal narrative guiding you through the meditation or self-hypnosis journey, or your inner self-talk taking you through these steps. Choose instrumental soundscapes that make you feel relaxed. I began experimenting with classical radio but found the adverts were appallingly inappropriate. Just as you're drifting into slumber, a piercing voice interrupts you to tell you about their supermarket offers.

So I ditched the radio stations and turned to sleep soundscapes on streaming services. There's a wide range to choose from. Some were not appropriate (just like some of the playlists described as '*for focus*' aren't) because although they were low volume and slow, they often contained irritating factors. For instance, a quiet and chilled piano piece seems from the outset to be conducive to sleep, but when one hand of the pianist repeatedly goes over and over the same phrase for prolonged periods, it becomes distracting and eventually irritating. I now use very sparse soundscapes that have hardly any activity in them at all. They're quite 'floaty'. They work really well for me and also provide a superb backdrop for guided journeys into a trance. Many people find that white noise, binaural, or monoaural playlists help transition them into sleep. There are many such playlists that are described as being designed to induce deep sleep delta brainwaves. I didn't use these approaches because I found other soundscapes that work well for me.

DIVE DEEPER

If you want to learn more about the science of sleep, read Matthew Walker's superb book and watch some of his talks on YouTube.

Why We Sleep by Matthew Walker

Chapter 8

Maintaining

Did you know the medical profession and the World Health Organisation are moving towards recognising ageing as a disease? It's preventable, not inevitable. Biohackers fully intend to live healthily to 100 years and beyond. I do too

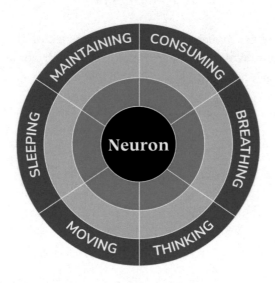

The previous chapters showed you what I did to fix and futureproof my own wellness. However, the key to living a long healthy life is maintaining these good habits. It's not enough to just do them for a few months. They have to become your forever habits. This chapter will show you the things I did to increase the likelihood that I'll maintain this lifestyle.

Let me first explain a few things that have helped drive my actions. I've seen the future, and it's definitely not a future I want to experience. A few years ago, I was invited by a leading over-50s brand to spend a week on their luxury cruise liner. There were a few hundred of their most loyal customers aged over 70 on board. I was dismayed at the sight of so many walking frames and wheelchairs. Most of the passengers were rather frail and infirm. Sadly, this group actually does quite accurately represent the health trends being seen in the general population. Our older adults have not been ageing well. They are living longer because medical science can keep them alive, but not in good health. The damage was done during their earlier adult life. It was driven by poor habits in their 30s, 40s, 50s, 60s but is now resulting in symptoms that impair their quality of life in their 70s, 80s, 90s and 100s. This is not the future I want, and I'm sure you don't either. Decades of poor health is not something to look forward to.

Spending several days immersed in this cruise ship environment was quite enlightening and somewhat depressing. I've also noticed my neighbourhood now has a care home on virtually every corner. Several beautiful old Victorian homes here have been turned into nursing facilities. Large 'super-homes' have also been built to try to cope with the rising demand of frail and infirm older adults. Even with increasing numbers of these premises, there's still a long waiting list if you need to find one and become a resident. Our ageing population has not aged well. It's not their fault. They are the result of many inventions and trends that happened in our society. I'd like to reduce the need for these facilities in future by showing younger generations how to age well. Success to me would be seeing these wonderful Victorian buildings being turned back into family homes. The hacks and habits I've used in my experiment could help ensure you live healthily to 100 or beyond. They are designed to reduce numerous risk factors that are known to cause preventable chronic diseases that are wrecking the lives of today's older adult population.

My formula is very straightforward. Everything I do falls into these three areas that I focused on:

1. Setting a rock-solid vision
2. Maintaining a rock-solid mindset
3. Establishing a rock-solid routine

If you nail those three things, you've significantly increased the likelihood that you'll enjoy good health, wealth and happiness throughout a long life. The concepts I've used in this book are at the more natural end of the biohacking approach. At the more extreme end, there is also a lot of fascinating stuff happening that will undoubtedly influence how we age – or don't – in future decades. The science of ageing (and anti-ageing) has become an enormous field worth hundreds of billions of dollars. There are already several supplements and procedures available to consumers. Youthfulness doesn't come from skin moisturisers. Those who are serious about it dive to a deep cellular level to achieve results. The aim is to slow, stop or even reverse the rate that your cells age. The hacks described earlier in this book are designed to remove things that are known to accelerate the ageing of your cells. For example, eliminating foods from your shopping lists that are known to cause insulin spikes in your bloodstream and inflammation in your cells; removing stressors that drive a repeated secretion of cortisol; removing toxins and waste products from your cells (and the area surrounding your cells) that accelerate the death of those cells or cause the halt of the regeneration of new cells.

As well as addressing lifestyle, it's now possible to use science to lend a helping hand. For example, Dave Asprey has had a full body stem cell makeover in recent years to rejuvenate his body's ability to maintain cell metabolism and cell function. There are less drastic anti-ageing options available in supplement form, such as resveratrol, NMN and metformin. Resveratrol and NMN help activate sirtuin genes that play a critical role in functions such as DNA repair. NMN boosts levels of NAD, a molecule found in all cells that helps create energy. By the age of 50, we have much lower levels of NAD. So NMN is believed to help boost it. Resveratrol uses the NAD supply as fuel to increase the activation of sirtuin genes and help maintain and sustain our capacity to repair and regenerate our cells. Resveratrol is also found in red wine, among other things. However, you'd have to drink a vineyard of it to get sufficient quantities, so don't think the glass with your evening meal is going to provide the sirtuin boost you're looking for. Metformin has been around for a long while as a drug to treat diabetes. However, it's now also considered a longevity drug due to its positive effects on our metabolic processes. I find this field fascinating, but I'm much more focused on addressing the lifestyle aspects that accelerate cellular ageing and cell death. If you can make changes to your daily behaviour that remove the damaging triggers, then you've already boosted your longevity without the need for extra supplementation. I feel the same way about the nootropics that are now widely available. These supplements target your brain function and are claimed to enhance memory, creativity and cognition. However, those are functions that can also be achieved using the hacks described throughout this book.

Ultimately, whatever way you choose to do it, the aim is the same: to help the natural process of autophagy, whereby cells clean themselves so they can continue to work at their best. The word autophagy actually means "self-eating". It's a crucial part of wellness, so damaged components within the cell don't result in the death of that cell. Intermittent fasting, for instance, is a straightforward way of encouraging autophagy. By entering this fasted state, and the stage of ketogenesis, you're reducing insulin and inflammation. Even if this book only teaches you how to break your addiction to processed sugar and carbohydrates, you'll have significantly boosted the ability of your brain and body to function to their maximum potential. Nutrition is crucial. Maintaining a constant clean level of energy and clarity can propel you to superhuman levels in terms of achievements in health, wealth and happiness.

The following pages outline the things I did to maximise my ability to maintain the transformative hacks and habits presented in previous chapters. There are many different uses and definitions of the term hack, biohack, body hack, brain hack, and life hack. For the purposes of this discussion, I view a hack as something (e.g. a technique, action, device or substance) that complements natural biological processes, with the aim of producing a highly efficient positive effect in the shortest time and with the least required effort. Hacks are shortcuts, designed to deliver maximum results with the minimum outlay. Habits, on the other hand, can produce positive or negative effects and can be highly inefficient. A hack can be something you do just once. Whereas a habit is something you do repeatedly over time. So, the key to success is learning the hacks and then embedding them into your life as positive habits. This process is a challenge in the early stages but ultimately becomes so automated that it's a breeze.

I believe that once you've achieved general good body health, age is simply a mindset. Aches and pains are often accepted by people as a "normal" part of ageing. They're not. If you have aches and pains, your body and brain are sending those signals to get your attention. Your biology is asking you to make some changes to fix the damage. If you didn't know your biological age and someone asked you how old you felt, what figure would you say? I'm now in my 50s, but I'd say late 20s or early 30s.

My Top Hacks For Maintaining

1. I measured my baselines

I love to measure and analyse things. I've been doing this throughout my professional career. Recording key information about the state of your health gives you extremely useful baselines. These can be used to maintain motivation towards goals, as benchmarks to compare yourself with other people in your age group, and to look for any unusual changes. I made a regular note of a range of scores, such as heart rate variability, resting heart rate, and weight. However, towards the end of my experiment, I also wanted to dive deeper and obtain a baseline measurement regarding the health status and biological age of my cells. One way of doing this is to measure the length of your telomeres. Telomeres are protective caps located on the ends of our chromosomes. Chromosomes are long pieces of DNA in our cells. DNA is the genetic code that contains the instructions for cells to grow and function. DNA is the blueprint of life. Imagine a chromosome as like a shoelace, and the telomeres are at each end to protect the shoelace from fraying. Cells repeatedly divide throughout life, but this cannot happen indefinitely. Telomeres also divide every time the cell divides. Eventually, the telomere becomes too short to be able to provide sufficient protection. This means the chromosomes will ultimately be unable to split correctly any further. The ends become too damaged, and information is lost. So, the telomeres are a bit like a molecular clock, counting down the lifespan and showing how many more times the cell can successfully divide. Telomere length shortens with age. It can also be accelerated by poor environmental and lifestyle factors because the cells have to divide and replicate more frequently to replace damaged cells. For those reasons, it's an interesting measure of biological age. I'm currently researching labs that offer this in the UK because the test I wanted is only available in North America at present.

I also obtained a measurement of my glycan activity as this is also considered a biomarker of biological ageing. Glycans are molecules of sugar that surround proteins in our body. They play an important role in our immune system by attaching to antibodies (Immunoglobulin G – IgG – is the most common) and modulate their activation, in particular by determining whether they are activated to play a pro-inflammatory or anti-inflammatory role. We need a balance of pro-inflammatory and anti-inflammatory glycans to keep inflammation in check. These molecules, therefore, are a useful marker of our general health status and our biological age. Interestingly, I discovered that the most dramatic changes in the glycan balance and inflammatory response happens in women between the age of 45 and 55. The hormonal changes during this decade can increase biological ageing by up to 30% and lead to disease. So, paying attention to my lifestyle, habits and environmental surroundings is particularly important for me right now in my 50s. My Glycan Age test result was 51. I was happy with that score because I'm fairly sure that a few years ago, it would have been older. So, my healthier daily habits are managing to bring my ageing process back into line with my chronological age. That's pleasing and motivating. Alarmingly, I apparently scored better than 68% of people. According to my post-test consultation, I discovered they commonly find that people aged mid-20s to mid-30s have a Glycan Age of mid-40s to 50s. This is due to poor lifestyle-driven inflammation accelerating the biological ageing of their cells. Now that I've brought my biological age back in line with my chronological age, I'm going to see how much more I can slow this ageing process in future years by continuing to keep inflammation in check. I'll recheck my test results annually to monitor how well my daily routines and eating habits are achieving this goal.

Of course, this sort of precision health isn't affordable for everyone. I spent almost £300 on the glycan test alone. My gut microbiome test was another £150, and the telomere test also runs into the hundreds. However, these aren't tests that I would have done regularly. They are simply ways to provide useful biomarker benchmarks that can help you maintain the motivation to live a healthy lifestyle.

2. I made sure limiting beliefs were totally gone

This actually turned out to be quite a big one for me. I hadn't even realised I had limiting beliefs, but once I dug down, they became apparent. These subconscious programmes run in the background of your mind without your awareness and can have a significant impact on how your life plays out. They can impact your health, wealth and happiness. Limiting beliefs can be erased, but you have to remove them at their deepest level. Think of it as weeds living in a grassy garden. You could mow over them, and the garden would look great for a while. But after a short time, they reappear because they were never really gone. To remove those weeds permanently, you have to dig down deep to make sure you remove every trace of their roots. The root causes of your limiting beliefs are experiences from your past. They're often so insignificant to your conscious mind that you'll have trouble finding them at first, but they are lurking there. I realised that I had limiting beliefs around wealth. Throughout my life, I have earned much higher sums than others in my peer group. However, my wealth goals were hitting a ceiling (a ceiling called limiting beliefs). In order to achieve financial freedom in our modern world, you need to build a significant amount of wealth. Earning a good salary is not the same as having financial freedom. If your job is lost or your business struggles, you are very quickly plunged into a highly stressful situation. The pandemic put many people, including me, in that situation. Income is not the same as financial wealth. Income can end suddenly, but your wealth can continue to support you. Stress about money problems damages your health and your happiness. It's one of the leading causes of stress in our modern society. I noticed that limiting beliefs based on my expertise also fed negatively into my limiting beliefs around wealth. These beliefs are often also experienced as an inferiority complex or imposter syndrome, whereby you don't fully push and promote yourself comfortably at the level you should. Through my bedtime self-hypnosis sessions, it became very apparent that these limiting beliefs around wealth and my ability were living in my subconscious. Once I removed them, I immediately began to notice wealth flowing towards me. Complete financial freedom is my new wealth goal, and it no longer has a ceiling. I realised that my previous wealth goal vision wasn't large enough and wasn't prioritised and addressed in sufficient detail. True wellness requires mastery of health, wealth and happiness - they're interlinked. You can't ignore one. If one is weak, all three are compromised. Find your limiting beliefs and use the approaches in previous chapters to eliminate them from your subconscious. Keep checking and refreshing them to maintain this robust approach and keep limiting beliefs at bay.

3. I strongly aligned vision with purpose

In order to turn your new habits into forever habits, it's hugely helpful to find ways of attaching them to a higher purpose, something that's really important to you. Think hard about what you want to achieve in life. Don't just trundle on, wasting each precious day. What matters to you? Why do you want to succeed in livi. long, healthy life? Is it so that you have more time w. your children? Is it so that you have more time to achieve some higher life purpose that you feel you're here to follow? What excites you, energises you, inspires you? What will get you out of bed every morning? Find the things that give you this sense of buzz. When I began my professional career in the early 1990s, I had a strong vision and enthusiasm, which was linked with my passion for teaching people how to improve their health and performance. Through various twists and turns throughout the decades, my professional life gradually drifted in a different direction. As I mentioned in earlier chapters, I became disillusioned with the "exercise and fitness" industry because it was clear in the 1990s that it was not a true route to wellness. I drifted into the events world mainly because I'd been using music in my health and wellness work, and it seemed fun. I began organising events for brands, using behavioural science principles to give customers a good time through music experiences. Don't get me wrong, I consider live music-driven social experiences to be extremely valuable, but they're not aligned with my vision or sense of purpose. I want to help people live healthier lives for longer. Organising a great live music event isn't going to help the general public fix their health. It also isn't the best use of my skills, experience and depth of knowledge. My events work wasn't making me leap out of bed every morning. So part of my experiment involved pivoting away from my event work and back towards my health and wellness work.

where I think I can contribute the most value to the
 ⅃. What contribution do you think you have to offer
 world? Are you actively delivering that contribution
 ⅃rough your work right now, or are you trundling along
in a job you don't enjoy because it's "easier" to keep
doing that than face the challenge of change? Life is short
(even if you live to 100). Make the most of it. Find your
passion, match it with your skills. Align your vision with
passion and purpose. You'll soon notice how your energy
levels supercharge and your health, wealth and happiness
all benefit. You'll have found a reason for maintaining
your new routine of habits.

4. I set goals for health, wealth and happiness

I saw a sketch today of two ladders side by side. The
ladder on the left had lots and lots of rungs, all very
closely and evenly distributed. The ladder on the right had
very few rungs, and they were spaced very far apart. The
person on the left ladder had climbed towards the top by
using all the rungs. However, the person holding the
ladder on the right was still at the bottom because s/he
couldn't reach the first rung. They were spaced out too far
and were out of reach. I loved this image. It perfectly
describes goal setting and is why people fail to continue
their good intentions regarding health (and wealth). They
have a goal, but it's far too large and distant. It's out of
reach because it's too complex or takes too long to
achieve. In most cases, it's actually not a goal; it's a
vision or a project, and therefore consists of a lot of goals,

not just one. The key to progressing up the ladder is taking small steps. There may be lots of rungs, but every time you successfully ascend to the next rung, you're closer to the end goal, and you get a little sense of achievement. That buzz is called dopamine, and it's the vital brain chemical if you want to succeed. In previous chapters, we mentioned that dopamine, norepinephrine (the brain's version of adrenaline) and acetylcholine work together to move you towards important things. Those three chemicals play a vital role in rewarding us for little successes, helping us to learn, remember and – most importantly – encourage us to continue the journey. As our key neuromodulator, dopamine in the reward system is vital. The little habits I embedded help to trigger little bursts of dopamine to keep me highly motivated and incentivised to continue. Small actions like making your bed really well in the morning, spending a few minutes on the gratitude journal and smelling the freshly brewed ground coffee all help trigger little secretions of dopamine to keep my neurons stimulated towards my goals.

Find your end goal and then break it down into much more achievable parts. "Launching a new business" is a very large undertaking and isn't specific enough to drive progress. "Improving my health" isn't specific enough either. You need to identify all the detail and map out the steps in the journey. Then start ticking them off. When my dog is covered in mud after a long walk through the fields, there are several steps to getting him clean. Trying to groom him with a small brush is not going to produce the end result I'm looking for. He's too covered in mud to get the comb through his fur. First, I need to hose the outer layer of mud off him. Then I need to shampoo and rinse him to get the remaining muck out of his fur. Then I need to wait for him to dry a little. NOW the brush will work well. I can finesse his final grooming and pop on his smart, clean collar, so he looks like a dog and is allowed back in the house again.

Goal-setting is a vital part of maintaining your new routine. This is why most of the hacks and habits I used took a short space of time. They are easy to tick off each day, but they move me towards the end goal of a lifelong healthy lifestyle. People who don't set intermediate goals get overwhelmed by the scale of the large goal. Break it down. I learnt the skill and power of goal-setting at a very young age in the sports world. I've used it every day throughout my whole life, and it's enabled me to reach many achievements.

5. *I focused intensely on routine*

From the outset of my experiment, I knew I needed to make the changes to my daily behaviour easy to maintain; they needed to be simple and short. They also needed to be highly repeatable. The brain learns through repetition. The aim is to repeatedly produce these habits regularly enough so the connections between the participating neurons are so strong this habit becomes automated. You're literally rewiring your brain. Most people give up and go back to their previous habits before the new habits are embedded strongly enough to erase their old unhealthy habits. I adopted a method called 'habit stacking' or 'habit chaining'. This approach can give you high levels of success for maintaining a new habit and quickly embedding it into your routine. You simply attach a new habit to an existing habit that's already deeply embedded. For example, I brew my pot of coffee every morning. Now when the coffee is brewing, I go into the lounge and do gratitude cuddles with my dog. If I had vowed to "do gratitude every morning", it's very doubtful that I would have continued doing it for long. Here's another example: I always let my dog into the garden first thing in the morning. Now I also accompany him outside, so I get early daylight in my eyes to set my suprachiasmatic nuclei master sleep timer. I'm merely using patterns of behaviours that have been firmly embedded through years of repetition (making a morning coffee and letting my dog outside) and linking new habits to them. Gradually I added more and more of my new habits into a longer chain. The key to success with habit stacking is choosing pre-existing practices (ones you want to keep) that are strong enough to attach other habits to. For instance, if I only occasionally let the dog out in the morning, it wouldn't have proven to be such a rock-solid foundation for stacking new habits on top of. The new habits soon became effortless. Because the patterns tended to happen at the same time of day, it also became easy for me to create a timed routine that maximised the effectiveness of the hacks. For example, if my habit of letting the dog outside happened at varying times through the morning, the "going outside" hack wouldn't have been as effective because it's based on getting natural light onto your retina as early as possible. Similarly, the habit I attached to my brewing coffee was gratitude. This doesn't need to have a time attached to it. So, it doesn't matter if my morning coffee happens at 6am or 11am. Whereas, if I'd attached my "going outside" hack to my coffee brewing instead of my dog, it wouldn't have been as effective because getting sun in your eyes at 6am is going to be more effective for a good night's sleep than doing it at 11am. Use strong positive habits that are already embedded into your daily routine (e.g. opening the curtains, brushing your teeth) as the anchor to build new habits. This technique is far easier to maintain than just trying to use sheer will power. My routine is laid out in detail in Part Two of this book. Repetition is vital in the early stages to accelerate the strengthening of the synaptic connections between neurons. The first 30 days are crucial.

6. I found like-minded friends who see my value

In some ways, this is related to the issue of limiting beliefs. I realised I needed to spend time – both in-person and online – with people who shared the same goals and views as me and also would recognise my value and support my efforts in my journey. So I joined several online groups around topics like biohacking, success mindset, and wealth goals. Even though these people were strangers, the positive effect of peer support is invaluable, particularly in the early days, when the journey is new and daunting. In fact, it can sometimes be much more useful to obtain regular peer support from people you don't know than from your friends and family. You will get high value from spending time with these groups. If you're only spending time with people who are unhealthy, it's likely you will remain unhealthy. Look around you and if you don't think you have the right support network, find a new one. It's simple to do that online these days. Find new groups that are strongly aligned with your new health, wealth and happiness goals. This will greatly increase your chance of success.

7. *I continued to fuel my interest*

Compared with the average person, I have a much greater depth of knowledge in the field of neuroscience and physiology principles. It's the result of a 30-year learning journey. However, that learning journey will never stop. I amassed new knowledge about the brain and body every day.

We actually still know very little about the brain because it's so complex. If you can ignite the flame of interest and become fascinated by your body and brain, you'll find that wellness becomes a fun and satisfying journey through life, rather than a chore. It can become your hobby as well as a habit.

I have always had an enduring fascination with the brain. It's truly incredible. I'm nowhere near the end of my learning journey. I fuelled my interest by reading lots of books on the subject, attending conferences and seminars about neuroscience and biohacking topics, watching hundreds of hours of talks and lectures online, and completing additional postgraduate applied neurobiology modules at the Institute of Neuroscience. The more I learn, the more fascinated I become.

I admit I'm more interested in the human brain and body than most people. However, I would urge you to start learning about it. The more you learn about your body and brain, the more likely it becomes that you will make the right choices about looking after it.

I called the approach throughout this book 'smart wellness' because it involves making educated decisions about your daily habits. Smart wellness is a bit like having an eye test. At first, when you're asked to read the distant letters, they're too blurry. Then, as the optician changes the lenses, the letters gradually become clearer until they are very sharply visible to you. Think of the experience of these lens changes as your journey through knowledge. At first, you don't know much about your body and brain, so you make mistakes. But as your increased knowledge accumulates, the right choices become clearer and clearer. Find the aspect of health that most interests you and learn more about it. Spending half an hour a day learning about how your brain and body work is more likely to bring greater long-term health benefits than half an hour doing inefficient exercises in a gym.

I'm currently fuelling my fascination by digging deeper into nutritional science. You know from previous chapters that the approach I used first was to break my supermarket habit and dramatically increase my daily intake of plant-based foods. Now I'm taking that a step further by examining the fruit and veg types in more detail. The Environmental Working Group releases an annual list of foods found to contain the highest and lowest traces of pesticides. In 2020, their "Dirty Dozen" (in order) were strawberries, spinach, kale, nectarines, apples, grapes, peaches, cherries, pears, tomatoes, celery and potatoes. Based on this list, I'm now trying to source organic providers of these items to reduce my exposure to toxins. The EWG also released a "Clean 15" that in 2020 featured (in order) avocados, sweetcorn, pineapple, onions, papaya, peas, eggplant, asparagus, cauliflower, cantaloupe melon, broccoli, mushrooms, cabbage, honeydew melon and kiwi fruit. So, I'm trying to focus my intake on those 15 clean items and away from the dirty dozen.

8. I added an extra layer of neuroplasticity

Since my PhD, I've become increasingly involved in the field of dementia. My research clearly showed that the music we're exposed to during our youth holds the key to maintaining a connection to someone who's locked in the confusing world of late-stage dementia. In these later stages, music becomes almost the only constant and is something that can pull them out of their world and back into ours for a short time as we share songs from their past together. At the time of the publication of my doctoral thesis in 2015, the value of music was not being extracted in dementia care. This was one of the findings of my research, even though it hadn't been one of my original areas of study. My post-doctoral work continued to explore this field of music and dementia. I contributed to several UK government groups examining this field and wrote a music strategy for the NHS's first 'dementia village'. In recent years I've also seen the impact of dementia on my own family and friends. I learnt that one-third of dementia cases could have been prevented by a healthier lifestyle during adulthood. This became a driving influence in my work and is one of the main reasons I set out to create a wellness programme. This book outlines hacks to help tackle most of the risk factors associated with brain degeneration. You've learnt how to reduce inflammation in your body by consuming the right things at the right time of day. You've learnt how to ensure stress chemicals aren't poisoning your system by using breathing, meditation, mindfulness and self-hypnosis. You've learnt how to achieve more effective movement without the need for more "exercise". You've learnt how to use light to get consistently high-quality sleep. You've learnt how to set goals to throw off limiting beliefs and reach for greater health, wealth and happiness. There's one more element that you'll notice in my daily habits: I make sure I learn new complex things every day. I've mentioned in previous chapters that if you don't tax your brain, the cells gradually deteriorate over time. This process happens even faster if your lifestyle and environment are unhealthy. The age-related decline of brain tissue is known as *negative plasticity* and can be seen in brain scans as gaping holes where neurons once were. This degeneration leads to impaired cognitive function – something that often gets brushed off as a "senior moment". Negative plasticity is not inevitable. It's also possible to not only maintain healthy brain cells as we age, but actually build new connections. The most effective way to do this is by learning new things. This is *positive plasticity*. Brains are constantly changing throughout life. Old connections between neurons are lost, and new ones are formed. Learning a musical instrument, a complex dance routine, or a language are highly effective ways of achieving this result. They make lots of regions of the brain work hard. People often say to me that they read a book or do a crossword puzzle to "give their brain a workout", but your brain is already very good at doing those familiar exercises. It's not as much of a workout as you might think. The brain quickly automates things that it's done many times before. This is an energy conservation method. For maximum effect, you need to do things you've never done before. The brain loves novelty. It doesn't have a pre-existing pattern of neuronal connections for the novel task or challenge you're presenting it with. It has to start from scratch. For example, learning a new language involves understanding complex grammar rules and a huge volume of new words that need to have meaning from your native language attached to them. There is a significant level of demand on the brain as it captures the new sensory information, applies rules and gets to work storing this new experience. I view science in a similar way. The complex terminology and detailed molecular formulas and relationships make my brain work hard. Regularly exercising your brain in this way helps maintain and build brain connections. Think of it as like depositing small amounts of money in your pension account. You'll be glad of it in future years. Studies have shown that building a cognitive reserve (a high level of healthy functioning neuronal connections) can pay dividends in later life. Your brain learns to find new routes even if dementia eventually starts to creep in and kill off cells in certain areas of your brain. Your brain health work over the years will have given it the capacity to rewire itself if it needs to. So, don't neglect plasticity in your daily routine. Make sure you learn lots of new, complex things throughout your entire life. Learn instruments, learn languages, learn about science.

9. I frequently reminded myself I have an ancient brain

You'll have noticed in several previous chapters that the autonomic nervous system cropped up frequently. Most of our poor health today is caused by our modern inventions confusing the heck out of this ancient survival system. Consequently, it needs a helping hand. Due to its bidirectional nature, you've seen that we're able to quite easily step in and influence it. When I started my experiment, it soon became clear that I was not giving my vagus nerve enough attention, and I certainly wasn't giving it enough training. In previous chapters, I showed you how I used breathing, and my resonance frequency breathing rate, to improve my vagal tone. The aim is to help ensure this complex nerve can maintain a healthy control over my fight/flight/freeze response. I included regular breathing practice sessions, but in addition, I stacked this practice onto other habits. So, for instance, while doing my daily gratitude cuddles with my dog, I'd use low and slow breathing. I also did it for a few minutes when I went outside to get early natural light in the mornings. I also did it when loading the dishwasher. At a neurobiological level, our nervous system is constantly evaluating our environment – think of it as a security check: it puts everything through a scanner to determine whether it's safe and can be allowed to continue or not. It's a complex interaction between our higher brain areas (the more evolutionary modern cortical regions) and our lower, more primitive regions in the limbic region and brain stem. This is a bidirectional flow of information travelling to and from our central nervous system and autonomic nervous system (the sympathetic nerve fibres and the parasympathetic nerve fibres such as the vagus nerve). We may notice that our heart starts beating faster in certain situations where our nervous system has perceived some sort of threat. Sometimes that threat is simply triggered when we're outside of our comfort zone. Breathing is not the only technique we can use to regulate our autonomic nervous system. As humans, we also have a system known as the *social engagement system*, which connects our face with our heart via a separate branch of the vagus nerve. This means that as well as our regular sensory information channels, we can also assess whether an environment is safe or not through facial expressions, vocalisation, listening and movements of the head. Therefore, engaging with others has a significant influence on the state of our autonomic nervous system. This natural system is often dysfunctional when people have experienced trauma and become highly sensitive to being around other people. On days during the pandemic lockdown when I began feeling things were becoming a little overwhelming, I strolled along to the local coffee shop, stood at a Covid-19 safe distance in the queue, chatted with those next to me, smiled a lot, and strolled home. This social engagement system is extremely powerful and fast-acting. I used this along with breathing to enlist the help of my vagus nerve to maintain a healthy mindset. Note that there is another vagal nerve state that is linked with our freeze response and shuts us down, and immobilises us in complete states of emergency. However, for the purposes of this book, we are focused on the safety (rest and digest) state of the parasympathetic vagus nerve.

10. I used music

You'll have noticed by now that my use of music and sound is a constant throughout this smart wellness approach. It's a versatile sensory input that we can easily manipulate to produce specific results. The fact that our brain uses vocalisation and listening to assess for safe environments opens valuable opportunities for wellness. Music that falls within the frequency range of the human voice and resembles the pace and tone of a calm human voice can help reassure our brain that everything is ok. These sounds help send safety signals to maintain a relaxed state. The sound vibrations of music are also received by the touch receptors on our skin. I also actually used some devices that specifically use calming sound vibrations fed directly onto the skin of the wrist. There are some interesting studies showing that singing to plants helps them grow. It's thought that the air vibrations may mimic a breeze and result in the development of stronger stems. I don't know if this is a verified effect or not, but I found it an interesting concept. However, there is a mass of peer-reviewed scientific research showing a multitude of positive health effects that music can deliver for humans. Below I've listed just a few examples from the *Oxford Handbook of Music & The Brain* (2019) demonstrating the value of adding more music to our life.

Music can:

- positively trigger the social engagement system (to help engage safety mode)
- boost brain development in children
- maintain brain health during adulthood (building cognitive reserve)
- improve memory function
- modulate emotions, mood and arousal
- boost social interactions
- block distractors to improve executive function and cognition
- assist in achieving desired brain states
- boost effort and motivation
- improve sleep
- assist movement timing in Parkinson's disease
- reduce anxiety in dementia

We know music has been bringing humans together for tens of thousands of years. It was a group social activity until we invented solo performances and private solo listening through headphones. It's entertaining but more than mere entertainment. It's a powerful asset when you use it with intent. I embed music throughout my day to help me achieve specific brain states and maintain motivation during moments of weakness. Find the soundscapes and songs that work for you and have them on standby.

I've markedly increased the amount of time I'm using music to drive neural plasticity. I used to play the guitar regularly, but my brain already knows how to do that. Even learning new songs doesn't really provide enough of a challenge. So, as part of my ongoing 'maintaining' work, I make sure I have a new and challenging learning programme embedded in my routine. Throughout the year, I learnt to perform basic skills on the drums, I learnt to play the core chords on the ukulele, and I'm currently learning how to play complex lead guitar solos. Next, I'll learn some complex techniques on the piano. I've also just ordered a brain stimulator to examine the claims that it can boost skill learning by 45%. It sits on top of your head like a headset and delivers electrical impulses intended to prime the neurons in the motor cortex before starting the skills training sessions (my music learning sessions). I'm intrigued to try this out.

DIVE DEEPER

Here are a few of my favourite books if you want to dig deeper into ageing science, neuroplasticity, music neuroscience and habit formation techniques.

Lifespan: Why we age and why we don't have to by David Sinclair, PhD

The Polyvagal Theory by Stephen Porges

Brain Rules for Baby by John Medina

The Organised Mind by Daniel Levitin

The Changing Mind by Daniel Levitin

What Doesn't Kill Us by Scott Carney

The Runaway Species by Anthony Brandt & David Eagleman

Livewired by David Eagleman

Adventures in Human Being by Gavin Francis

Grit by Angela Duckworth

Tiny Habits by BJ Fogg

Atomic Habits by James Clear

The Art of Happiness by The Dalai Lama

Think Like A Monk by Jay Shetty

The Buddha and the Badass by Vishen Lakhiani

Extra Time by Camilla Cavendish

Music and Your Brain by Daniel Levitin

The Oxford Handbook of Music & the Brain edited by Michael Thaut and Donald Hodges

Sapiens by Yuval Noah Harari

Homo Deus by Yuval Noah Harari

PART TWO

My New Daily Routine
(forever)

SMART WELLNESS

Daily Habits

MORNING (from 0600)
These habits prime brain & body chemicals for a great day and great night's sleep

- Make your bed really well and acknowledge it
- Get early natural outdoor light in eyesight
- Make great coffee or tea and savour the taste and smell
- Write in your gratitude journal
- Learn something new and complex
- Outdoor walk (with steep incline), sea swim, or slow motion strength moves
- Contrast shower – hot to cold

WORKING DAY (from 0900)
These habits help the brain focus and keep stress chemicals low

- Make a to do list
- Divide tasks into chunks
- Use focus music playlists
- Turn on upbeat music for energy boosts
- Take short breaks frequently & move
- Attend virtual meetings to get some social contact
- Eat within an 8-hour window and drink water often
- Take a break for some low and slow breathing practice
- Soften your gaze and look away from your computer screen every hour

EVENING (from 1830)
These habits prime the brain chemistry for rest, repair and memory consolidation

- Get outside, take a walk and enjoy your surroundings
- Socialise with others
- Chill (e.g. TV, read, music, shower, bathe, exercise, play)
- Write down any incompletes that need to be addressed tomorrow
- Use dimmed low level light and avoid screens (or use blue blocker glasses)
- Switch on low volume, low tempo music
- Get into bed and listen to some guided meditation or self-hypnosis recordings

The following pages present my new daily routine, featuring the habits I complete every day. It's not a rigid, stressful schedule. I'm quite relaxed about it. If I miss something on some days, it's not the end of the world. I just try to make sure I don't miss it again the next day. From the outset of my experiment, I knew that it was essential to make this routine simple and enjoyable. The aim was to have a simple and automated range of habits that result in optimal and ongoing wellness.

Having this list greatly helped me maintain these habits early on, while I was eliminating previous poor routines. As you saw in previous pages, I used habit stacking as my technique of choice due to its ease and effectiveness. The habits on the following pages are hacks intended to use scientific principles to assist specific neurobiological or biological processes. They all are believed to increase the likelihood of neurons being stimulated (or not) in beneficial ways by the secretion of certain neurochemicals and hormones. I tend to more or less do them in the order they are shown due to how I stacked them and the function they are designed to affect. They worked for me, and they may work for you. Still, these are not medical recommendations – as with all health-related activity, please consult with your doctor if you think you may have underlying conditions that could be affected by any of the habits here. Good luck.

My Daily Habits & Hacks

Morning	Working Day (0930 – 1830)	Evening
Sync health measurements (Sleep cycles, RHR, HRV, RSA)	'To-Do' list (start with ticking off a few "incompletes")	Socialising
Make bed well	Use music/soundtracks as required	TV/reading/internet
Stand outside	Meetings - pm	Dog walk
Make (and smell) great coffee mindfully	Panoramic gaze & breathing practice	Jot down any 'incompletes' that are on my mind
Practice gratitude	Eating in an eight-hour window	Dimmed low lights and bedtime oil
Learning (motor and cognitive)	Dog Walk / sea swim	Low volume chilled music
Shower (hot to cold)	Additional exercises e.g. slow-motion strength	Self-hypnosis / breathing

Chapter 9

Morning Routine

Morning (0600 start)
Wake-up routine:
Make bed really well
Stand outside for bright natural light
Make a great pot of coffee
Practice gratitude
Slow-motion moves and stretches
Learning new things:
Reading, researching, writing (cognitive)
Guitar learning (motor)

<u>Habit 1 – Make your bed really well</u>
(approx. 3 mins)

Getting an early boost of dopamine and serotonin sets you up for a great day. Self-rewards can trigger the release of these chemicals in your brain, even for just little achievements like doing a great job of bed-making. Simply take a few minutes to relax and breathe low and slow while making your bed really well. Then stand back and acknowledge your effort. You don't have to congratulate yourself out loud. Just visually enjoy the sight of your tidy bed. It may sound unlikely, but this is a fast and easy way to initiate an early kick of positive neurochemicals and engage the parasympathetic nervous system. I also found a red blanket to cover the duvet. It makes the bed making process even more satisfying because it looks so smooth when done well.

<u>Habit 2 – Stand outside to get early daylight</u>
(approx. 5 minutes)

Cortisol and melatonin chemicals operate in cycles that are greatly influenced by the light to which our eyes are exposed. It's imperative to maintain this rhythm by giving your brain the natural light levels it needs at the right time of the day.

The cells in the retina have low sensitivity in the morning, so ideally you need to go outside because indoor light is too weak to deliver the same effect as natural light. Stand in your garden or doorway or open a window and absorb the morning light. Don't look directly into the sun. I practice relaxed deep breathing for a few minutes while doing this to engage the parasympathetic nervous system. Tune your mind into the natural sounds around you (unless your environmental sounds are negative, such as traffic).

Habit 3 – Make a great pot of coffee
(approx. 10 mins)

Again, this self-reward is a fast and simple way to release some dopamine and serotonin in your brain. For my first cup of coffee each day, I use high-quality, expensive coffee beans as a treat. This makes the whole process even more enjoyable and something worth getting out of bed for. They smell and taste amazing, and I look forward to them so much that it also helps me get out of bed at 6am instead of lying there, pressing the snooze button as I used to. I pay attention to every step and try to make a great brew. Then I congratulate my effort during the reward of the first savoured sniff and sip (sometimes with my inner voice and sometimes out loud).

I used to have a coffee machine that required me to put in a pod and press a button. I realised that this wasn't maximising the potential value that can be extracted from a morning coffee ritual. Instead, I began to use a coffee grinder and a filter coffee machine. The smell and sound of the coffee-making process became much more intensified and satisfying.

Habit 4 – Practice gratitude
(approx. 5-10 minutes)

While the coffee is brewing, I sit with my dog, give him highly attentive cuddles and tell him how grateful I am for him. I breathe low and slow and say these things out loud. He loves this routine, and so do I. He loves it so much that as soon as he hears the coffee percolating, he now runs to the sofa and lies excitedly awaiting our gratitude cuddles. I tell him about lots of things I'm grateful for: the health and love of my family and friends; my warm, safe home; my happiness and success; my coffee; exciting, positive progress towards my goals; sunshine; my garden and more. I repeat many of the same things each day, and that doesn't matter. It's the practice of gratitude, not the specific items, that bring the benefits. With low, slow breathing, this is another easy way to engage the parasympathetic nervous system. If you don't have a pet, find another way to embed this practice into your routine (e.g. sitting in a favourite chair and writing in a journal).

Gratitude is a fascinating research topic currently attracting increasing neuroscience interest due to the visible changes to the brain and many aspects of wellbeing. It helps put larger stressors into perspective when you spent a bit of time reminding yourself of good things in your life and the wider world.

Habit 5 – Slow motion muscle moves and stretches
(approx. 10 mins)

Remember that muscle tissue naturally declines with age unless it is frequently overloaded. Maintaining muscle mass is vital to stemming or slowing this atrophy and keeping your body strong and in good health. Slow-motion moves efficiently bring muscle groups to exhaustion, so the adaptive response is triggered, and glycogen stores are depleted. This means it's a workout in just a few minutes. Flexibility is necessary, too, so I include a few basic stretching and breathing moves.

Habit 6 – Learn something new
(I spend up to 2 hours on this, but even 15 mins works)

Just as muscle tissue decays with age unless you exercise it, brain tissue experiences the same decline unless you actively prevent it. Plasticity, the rewiring of brain connections between neurons, requires a level of alertness and arousal followed by concentrated focus. This state is facilitated by the release of norepinephrine, acetylcholine and dopamine. Neurons involved in the period of deep focused work and learning are marked during activation. Deep rest periods later that night (during delta brainwave slow-wave sleep stages) feature a consolidation process where the neurons marked during the learning activity are consolidated into memory. Every morning I learn new things to boost the plasticity of my brain. This improves memory and helps nourish the nervous system tissue that's essential for brain cells to communicate with each other. Reading, researching and guitar tuition boosts my thinking and motor skills. I choose complex material that taxes me and presents me with words, formulas and movements that are unfamiliar. The effort and small goals drive norepinephrine and dopamine release even when I'm not quite nailing the techniques. I've also recently discovered that dopamine also acts as a buffer for norepinephrine, helping you to continue the effort for longer. Choose material and activities that your brain finds novel and challenging to see the most significant benefits. If you're feeling the frustration that often accompanies these early learning stages, you can be reasonably sure your brain is busy building new neural connections.

Chapter 10

Work-Day Routine

Working Day (0930 – 1830)
Work routine:
Music on
Tasklist (using focus runway)
Meetings / virtual meetings
Breaks:
Panoramic gaze
Eating
Breathing practice
Walk/sea swim

Habit 7 – Turn on some music

As detailed in my previous book, *The Music Diet*, one of the fastest ways to get into the right mindset and release important brain chemicals is by turning on some music. I use calming soundscapes for focus early in the day and higher energy songs in the afternoon when I need a boost. This helps the drip-feed of brain chemicals that are involved in feelings of safety, positivity and happiness. Some of my life goals often seem distant, unachievable and overwhelming, so I find that music is a life-saver when it comes to reaching for a hack to lift me out of a funk when a setback or rejection has occurred. Don't underestimate the power of music. It's a highly effective asset within your mindset toolkit. It can very quickly flip you from sympathetic stress response mode to parasympathetic relaxation mode (even when you just hum the songs or play them silently in your mind), particularly when combined with breathing practice.

Habit 8 – Break up focus tasks into chunks
(approx 20 min per session with 5 mins breaks)

The working day is when the sympathetic nervous system (alert system) might start to dominate and elevate cortisol levels (the stress chemical). A systematic approach to workload is essential in order to remain in control of the autonomic nervous system. Make to-do lists and split tasks into smaller chunks to keep the autonomic nervous system in check. Some jobs require a lot of concentration. As you learned previously, this cognitive effort involves a cocktail of brain chemicals, such as acetylcholine, norepinephrine and dopamine. It's also necessary to switch to task-oriented regions of the brain, such as the pre-frontal cortex, and away from the default mode network to prevent your mind from wandering. I also use a specially designed soundscape called the Focus Runway to help keep my brain focused. I also fix my eyes fully on the visual target of the Focus Runway rotating brain for a minute or so on screen before starting the task. This releases acetylcholine and helps transition into the work. If I find that my mind drifts off the task, I repeat the process until I'm deeply immersed again.

Habit 9 – Engage in meetings

We're not designed to spend long periods alone. Meeting, talking to and collaborating with others (even just through virtual meetings) boosts the release of oxytocin, our social hormone, plus serotonin and dopamine as we smile during conversation and enjoy feelings of progress towards goals. However, too many unnecessary meetings (or meetings that are too long or perceived as threatening) can increase your stress hormone. They eat into your time, leaving less for staying on top of your to-do list. The inability to keep up with a workload is a leading cause of work-related stress, so be brutal about your diary and don't let people overload you with unnecessary meetings. Employers should be particularly aware of this issue now that remote working is the norm post-pandemic.

Habit 10 – Practice peripheral gaze
(2 mins)

It's imperative to frequently break away from the desk and computer screen throughout the day and regain control over your cortisol levels and autonomic nervous system. The visual system is connected via nerve tissue to the autonomic nervous system and parts of our emotional limbic system (especially the amygdala). A few minutes of peripheral gaze practice can make the brain aware that there are no immediate threats in our vicinity. This relaxed focus combined with low and slow breathing through the nose (see Step 11) can quickly switch our autonomic nervous system from the sympathetic network (alert mode, stress response) back into parasympathetic mode (relax mode) and keep cortisol under control. This is a fast and useful technique that's easy to use anywhere. To switch to peripheral vision, simply relax your focus so you can see everything within your visual field to the left and right without moving your head or eyes. It's a bit like panoramic mode on your camera. Once you get the hang of it, you'll find it easy.

Habit 11 – Practice breathing
(5-20 min sessions)

Most of us are not breathing correctly. Train yourself to always breathe through your nose. Your nasal passages release nitric oxide, so inhaled air molecules collect this chemical and transfer it into your bloodstream via the lungs. Nitric oxide helps lower blood pressure. Your nose contains the hair cells and mucous designed to purify the air and warm it to the right temperature before it reaches the lungs. Breathing through your mouth exposes your lungs to unfiltered air, and is linked to gum disease. A few low and slow nasal breaths (using the diaphragm muscle, not the chest) triggers a fast relaxation response by engaging the parasympathetic nervous system. Breathing correctly by engaging the diaphragm also helps keep food moving along its internal journey through our intestines. A few mins of breathing practice regularly throughout the day will help you embed low and slow nasal breathing as a default technique, giving you a fast route to relaxation and cortisol control.

If you're feeling particularly stressed and overwhelmed, try a physiological sigh. Inhale and then quickly inhale in a bit more air before exhaling slowly. This double inhale snaps open and fills air sacs to their capacity, rapidly enabling oxygen to enter the bloodstream and lots of carbon dioxide to be removed during the long, slow exhale. This assists in triggering a relaxation response because raising carbon dioxide in the bloodstream is part of the stress signalling response. A physiological sigh can help you quickly reset oxygen and carbon dioxide levels and tells your autonomic nervous system that there is no threat to respond to.

Habit 12 – Eating during an eight-hour window

The brain needs an enormous amount of fuel. It weighs only about 2% of our total body weight but burns approximately 20% of our daily energy consumption. However, most of us are eating too much food, the wrong food, and at the wrong time of day. I aim to consume my meals within an eight-hour eating period, letting my body fast during the other 16 hours. It's very easy to do once you get into the habit. Push your breakfast to later in the morning and eat earlier in the evening. I ditched processed sugar and high carbohydrate food, and focused on vegetables, fish and lean white meat as much as possible. Your brain needs essential fatty acids, so I consume plenty of omega-3 rich food such as salmon and walnuts. I get my sugar fix from fruit (but in moderation) and dark chocolate. I also drink as much water as I can throughout the day, as this has a considerable impact on brain function. If your BMI is above the healthy limit, your brain's biological age increases by approximately 10 years. This statistic should terrify you into addressing poor eating and drinking habits and embedding brain exercises and sleep into your daily routine to reverse the damage.

Habit 13 – Practice brainwave training
(15-20 mins)

The brain operates on electrical impulses being passed from neuron (brain cell) to neuron. When they are highly active, they emit a different frequency than when we're relaxed or asleep. During waking and working hours, brainwaves are predominantly beta waves, but it's useful to be able to slow them into more alpha and theta waves on command when we want to relax. This is called *entrainment* and can be developed by using mindfulness, meditation, self-hypnosis or breathing practices. I sometimes use a headband that can measure brainwaves in real-time while I practice controlling them. I use a heart rate monitor that shows me how my autonomic nervous system is responding. The HRV provides a useful indicator of the health of my parasympathetic nervous system due to my breathing and mind state training practices. Tech tools like this are helpful because they make practice more fun and meaningful, and help you see what techniques work best for you. I also often use soundscapes for these sessions.

Habit 14 – Walk and/or sea swim
(15-45 mins)

Moving is good for us. Interestingly, moving forward through our environment may also trigger a relaxation response on top of the general exercise benefits, due to the way brains processes forward motion through optic flow. Several studies have examined the link between these eye movements and the part of our brain that plays a central role in our anxiety responses, the amygdala. Consequently, outdoor activities that incorporate forward self-motion such as walking, cycling, running and swimming could deliver additional relaxation benefits (they're better than doing the same activities on an indoor stationary exercise machine), due to the downregulation of the amygdala caused by the eye movements triggered by forward movement through the landscape. Plus, you get the added benefit of natural light exposure, which is important for vitamin D levels and circadian timer calibration. Listen to the natural sounds of the environment or a music playlist or podcast to help you move for longer.

Chapter 11

Evening Routine

Evening
Leisure, play and chill time:
Socialising
TV / reading / internet
Dog walk
Incompletes list
Bedtime routine:
Dimmed low lights
Low volume chilled music
Self-hypnosis/breathing
Sleep (by 11pm at the latest)

Habit 15 – Socialise / Play / Fun

Being in the presence of friends and family in positive social settings stimulates the release of social bonding chemical oxytocin, as well as the mood and motivation chemicals serotonin and dopamine. Incorporating play activities into this social experience increases the health benefits. However, frequently coupling your social activity with alcohol consumption somewhat destroys the benefits. Drinking alcohol compromises your sleep quality, leading to serious health defects. If drinking alcohol is essential to your social activity, try and do it at least four hours before bedtime. Alcohol entering your bloodstream immediately destroys the chemical balance. It quickly shuts down areas of the brain by turning on the release of GABA (the brain's "stop" neurochemical), then turns off the glutamate supply (the brain's "go" neurochemical) by blocking the receptors. Even small amounts of alcohol consumed frequently will gradually damage your brain as well as causing chaos in other areas of the body and your waistline. I aim to incorporate lots of social activity into my evenings but try not to make them all linked to alcohol consumption. For example, early evening dog walks with friends are an excellent way to switch off from work and for socialising while clocking up more steps.

Habit 16 – Chill

Doing nothing is as important to good health as taking action and doing something. We need a balance of both in order to control our ability to switch between being alert when necessary and relaxed when action is not required. Being able to switch off and "chill" becomes harder when the stress chemical cortisol has been allowed to dominate your existence. Cortisol should naturally fall as you approach bedtime. This effect is mirrored by a corresponding rise in melatonin to make you drowsy. As part of my chill routine, I often write a list of 'incompletes', things I didn't complete today, but I know need to be attended to tomorrow. It's important to get these out of your head and onto a list so your brain is no longer concerned about them. Then I try and lose myself in a good book, film, music, hypnotic trance, or meditation every evening. Chilling can take many forms. For some, it might just be sitting in the garden, having a lovely bath or a massage. Make your evenings conducive to relaxation. It doesn't matter what your favourite chill activity is. What matters is that you try and add a little chill time to your daily existence.

Habit 17 – Dim the indoor lights

At the start of the day, the light receptors at the back of your eyes have low sensitivity, so they need lots of bright natural light to set the melatonin and cortisol timers (see Step 2). But by evening, the cells are highly sensitive. Even a small amount of light can activate them. Indoor light is far too bright for these cells at night time. It's critical to make sure that indoor lights are dimmed in the evening and preferably positioned at a level below the eye line, so they are not shining down from above and mimicking the sun (e.g. table level lamps or floor lamps). Getting natural outdoor light at dusk can also help the brain know that sleep time is approaching. It has a different consistency to light earlier in the day. There are much lower levels of blue light at sunset than earlier in the daytime. Flooding your eyes with bright indoor artificial light (and high-level light such as ceiling lights) in the evening and late at night confuses your brain because it cannot tell if it's day time or night time. This type of light (and light from screens) emit much more blue light than the brain should be experiencing at the end of the day if it was in a natural environment. If you just can't put down your phone, buy a power timer plug that kills the electrical supply to your Wifi router at a certain time each night. If you really cannot break your evening screen habit, use blue light blocking glasses.

Habit 18 – Put on low volume chilled music

Just as loud, lively music can help boost energy levels and motivation earlier in the day, low volume relaxing music can help calm your brain and body ready for sleep. Use it as a background soundscape to set the scene for bedtime. Synchronise your low and slow breathing to the slow beat of the music to dial down brainwaves and engage the parasympathetic nervous system. Simple instrumental music is particularly good as it gives your brain less information to process and is less distracting. Let the music envelop you and create a sleep ambience. When done regularly with the same soundtrack, it can produce a priming effect, linking the sounds with sleep. I also place a few drops of an essential oil sleep scent on my pillow to further embed that association with sleep mode.

Habit 19 – Immerse in self-hypnosis / meditation
(approx. 20 mins)

The trance-like state of hypnosis is relatively easy to guide yourself into with practice, and it can deliver impressive rewards. There are many free, guided sessions online. Slowing your breathing and brainwaves in this way gradually takes you into a sleep state. However, during the journey, you pass through periods where you can have a strong connection with your unconscious mind. These are moments where it's possible to focus your mind on things you'd like to achieve in life. Build your focus, purpose and direction in life by telling your mind what you want. Don't underestimate how powerful this can be. Hypnosis produces a fascinating and unique brain state whereby you can simultaneously achieve deep focus and deep rest and relaxation. This delivers exceptional opportunities to achieve plasticity and learning and for shaping your beliefs and abilities. Pop your earphones in when you get into bed and make this hypnotic trance journey a regular part of your standard runway into sleep.

<u>Habit 20 – Sleep</u>
(7-9 hours of good quality sleep)

We now know that the brain doesn't "go to sleep". When our conscious mind is asleep, the brain is still at work, consolidating memories, removing toxins built up during the day and thoroughly restoring the body ready for action tomorrow. Lack of quality sleep over a prolonged period is now shown to be linked with degenerative brain diseases. The damage often builds over the decades and doesn't become visible until symptoms eventually appear much later. Sleep is essential to good health, so don't deprive yourself. Sleep scientists believe the adult brain needs seven-nine hours of good sleep each night in order to function well. This is something that few people consistently manage to achieve. If you cycle through five quality 90 min sleep cycles, that's 7.5 hours of sleep. That's what I aim for. Don't undo all the good health practices in the daytime by neglecting this final and critical piece of the jigsaw at night. The steps earlier in the day should prime you for a great night's sleep. Stick with the routine, and gradually you'll notice the impact on your sleep quality and your overall health.

None of us can guarantee our future good health, but all the daily habits aim to help you reduce risk factors and increase the chance of a good long, healthy, happy life with lots of great sleep. You might not think of sleep as a habit, but if you go to bed and get up at the same time each day, it does become an embedded habit.

Final Thoughts

Thanks for taking the time to read this book. It's covered a lot of ground. I've deliberately tried to avoid getting too detailed. I've also excluded some things in an attempt to make a vast and hugely complex subject easily consumable. I've aimed to give lots of examples, showing how I myself used these scientific principles in my everyday life to boost my own wellness.

My current health scores, and the transformation in my own health since I began this experiment, demonstrate that this Smart Wellness approach can have significant beneficial effects. I hope you experience the same success.

As I write this final note there are already changes taking place in the UK Government that reflect the increasing attention these facts are attracting. A new Office for Health Promotion will increase the focus on prevention rather than cure. It already recognises that the way we approach and promote healthy lifestyles is flawed and hasn't worked. The population is generally confused about nutrition (and/or being fed misleading information on packaging) and is frequently directed into exercise focused programmes that result in lack of progress (in relation to weight loss) and despondency. We need to get the correct information into the hands of the wider population if we are to succeed in finally achieving healthy nations. It's essential that we successfully break the addictive food and drink habits that are poisoning and suppressing our amazing in-built natural wellness systems.

In 2022, my final book in this Health Trilogy, titled *'Autotune'*, will detail what almost certainly is going to be the future of health, driven by simple and available biological tests informing personalised shopping lists and nutrition. This science and tech is already easily available to consumers. I'm using it myself for my own nutrition and that of my clients. I'm also on the cusp of launching a collaboration that will offer this level of bespoke service to a broader audience. Once this level of personalised, biological, data driven service becomes affordable to all it will have a huge impact on health and wellness. It is probably also the key to considerably extending healthy life expectancy. I look forward with excitement to the future developments in this field as I continue to research and refine my own approach in my quest for a healthy life to 100(+).

REMEMBER

Look after your neurons and they will look after you

SOURCE MATERIALS AND REFERENCES

The recommended reading and specific source materials that informed my approach to my wellness and the development of this Smart Wellness programme are listed at the end of each chapter.

If your interest has been ignited, and you'd like to explore additional deeper reading, as well as the latest scientific insights (since the original publication of this book), search your keyword of interest at these websites:

pubmed.ncbi.nlm.nih.gov

nature.com

cell.com